Healthy & Safe Homes

RESEARCH, PRACTICE, & POLICY

EDITORS

Rebecca L. Morley, MSPP
Angela D. Mickalide, PhD, CHES
Karin A. Mack, PhD

American
Public Health
Association

APHA

PRESS

www.aphabookstore.org

WASHINGTON, D.C. • 2011

American Public Health Association
800 I Street, NW
Washington, DC 20001-3710
www.apha.org

Georges C. Benjamin, M.D., F.A.C.P., *Executive Director*
Judith C. Hays, Ph.D., R.N., *Publications Board Liaison*

Printed and bound in the United States of America
Interior Design and Typesetting: Vanessa Sifford and The Manila Typesetting Company
Cover Design: Jennifer Strass
Printing and Binding: Victor Graphics, Inc.

Library of Congress Cataloging-in-Publication Data

Healthy and safe homes : research, practice, and policy / editors, Rebecca Morley, Angela Mickalide, and Karin A. Mack; foreword by Georges C. Benjamin.
    p. ; cm.
  Includes bibliographical references and index.
  ISBN-13: 978-0-87553-197-7 (alk. paper)
  ISBN-10: 0-87553-197-0 (alk. paper)
  1. Housing and health. I. Morley, Rebecca. II. Mickalide, Angela. III. Mack, Karin A. IV. American Public Health Association.
  [DNLM: 1. Housing—standards. 2. Family Health. WA 795 H434 2011]
  RA770.H437 2011
  613'.5—dc22

                        2010016765

ISBN 13: 978-0-87553-197-7
ISBN 10: 0-87553-197-0
10/2010

Table of Contents

Foreword

The publication of *Healthy and Safe Homes: Research, Practice, and Policy* marks an exciting advance in the effort to ensure that people across all socio-economic levels have access to healthy and affordable housing. All families should have quality, affordable housing; it serves as a foundation for a prosperous life. I welcome the publication of this book as one that provides practical tools and information to make the connection between health and housing conditions relatable to everyone.

This new book brings together perspectives of noted scientists, public health experts, housing advocates, and policy leaders to fully explain the problem of substandard housing that plagues our nation and offer holistic, strategic, and long-term solutions to fix it. The many experts who have contributed to this book lay out smart approaches to help achieve the goal of making healthy housing accessible to all. Expanding access to healthy and affordable housing is a first step to creating a country of healthier people.

With the ever-changing real estate market and recent housing booms and busts that many families in America have endured, most caregivers today feel lucky just to provide a roof over their children's heads and don't realize that living in substandard housing brings long-term consequences, or that it can lead to serious health problems, including asthma, allergies, developmental disabilities, lead poisoning, physical injuries, and cancer.

Substandard housing conditions are unequally distributed, with children of color and low-income families shouldering the majority of the burden. As a result, unhealthy housing contributes to our nation's disparities in health, failing schools, and even our over-populated juvenile justice system, adding further to the enormous and costly toll on our nation's health care system. The materials and tools gathered in this book clearly demonstrate that providing a roof is just part of the equation. All families in America need and deserve access to a *healthy* home where they can grow, thrive, and achieve.

This book incorporates perspectives from diverse fields to explain and present the scope of the problem of substandard housing. It makes a compelling case that comprehensive healthy housing requires the combined efforts of many public and private stakeholders—developers, investors, health professionals, government officials, leaders of community-based nonprofits and others—working toward a common goal.

The authors begin by explaining the connection between the home environment and personal health in a way that the public can understand and appreciate. From there, the book draws on scientific evidence and methodology to offer an action plan. Because the current means of addressing poor-quality housing is narrow in approach and therefore ineffective, despite the good intentions of the individuals involved, the book navigates previously uncharted territory by showing that healthy homes are only truly attained by first bringing together many diverse partners united by a common investment in creating a healthier society.

"Healthy housing" is influenced by a complex mix of interconnected issues that extend beyond each individual home. The book promotes integrating fields that typically operate in isolation such as public health, urban planning, air and water quality, building science, home safety, and social policy as necessary steps to advancing healthier housing.

Far too many children begin life disadvantaged because of the homes and neighborhoods in which they live. If we hope to improve the health of our families and our communities, we must give people living in poverty the opportunity to move up and out through a mix of affordable housing options, access to jobs, and social support. *Healthy and Safe Homes: Research, Practice, and Policy* is an important addition to the effort to draw attention to the role that substandard housing plays in perpetuating the cycle of poverty and its impact on human health. It is this perspective that guides the practical solutions presented in the chapters that follow as an understandable action plan to close the gap and improve the health of all.

Georges C. Benjamin, MD, FACP, FACEP (Emeritus)
Executive Director
American Public Health Association
Washington, DC

About the Authors

Grant Baldwin, PhD, MPH – Dr. Baldwin became Director of the Division of Unintentional Injury Prevention (DUIP) at the National Center for Injury Prevention and Control (NCIPC) in September 2008. Dr. Baldwin joined NCIPC in November 2006 as acting deputy director. Before this appointment, Dr. Baldwin served as a senior advisor in the Coordinating Center for Environmental Health and Injury Prevention and the National Center for Environmental Health (NCEH) Agency for Toxic Substances and Disease Registry (ATSDR). Dr. Baldwin received his PhD in health behavior and health education at the University of Michigan School of Public Health in 2003. He also received a MPH in behavioral sciences and health education from the Rollins School of Public Health at Emory University in 1996.

Mary Jean Brown, ScD, RN – Dr. Brown has been the Chief of the Lead Poisoning Prevention Branch at the CDC since 2003 and also is an adjunct professor of Society, Human Development, and Health at the Harvard School of Public Health. Dr. Brown received a ScD from the Harvard School of Public Health in 2000. She is a registered nurse who has been working in the area of childhood lead poisoning prevention for more than 25 years. During that time she became convinced that housing has a substantial impact on health and that the health of residents should be considered in all phases of housing construction, maintenance, and renovation.

Shane Diekman, PhD, MPH – Dr. Diekman is a behavioral scientist in the DUIP at the NCIPC. Dr. Diekman joined DUIP in 2004, with the primary responsibility of conducting research and implementing programs to reduce unintentional injuries around the home. His research focuses on designing and evaluating health promotion programs aimed at reducing health disparities, and his areas of interests include residential fires, falls among older adults, and alcohol use. Before coming to CDC, Dr. Diekman worked at the University of North Carolina Highway Safety Research Center, where he conducted behavioral science research and evaluation. Dr. Diekman earned his PhD in health behavior and health education at the University of North Carolina at Chapel Hill School of Public Health in 2004. His MPH in behavioral science and health education is from the Rollins School of Public Health at Emory University in 1996.

Annie Feighery, MPA, EdM – Ms. Feighery is a policy fellow and doctoral candidate in health education at Columbia University Teachers College. She earned a BA in anthropology and the University Honors Degree from the University of Texas at El Paso, an MPA in environmental science and policy from the Columbia University School of International and Public Affairs, and an EdM in international educational development from Columbia University Teachers College. Currently, Ms. Feighery is conducting research on maternal survival and social capital in global health.

Jerry Hershovitz, BA – Mr. Hershovitz retired from the CDC in January 2006 as acting associate director for Program Development, NCEH and ATSDR. Throughout his career he served in key management positions in programs that included childhood lead poisoning prevention, rodent control, and injury epidemiology and control. Mr. Hershovitz played a major role in the development and implementation of CDC's national strategy to revitalize the environmental public health services system. He was the architect of CDC's national healthy homes and integrated pest management initiatives and served as a consultant to the European office of the World Health Organization on issues related to healthy housing and vector management.

CDR Mark Jackson, USPHS, BS, REHS – CDR Mark Jackson, USPHS, is a public health advisor for the CDC's NCIPC. In this role he serves as the sole project officer for the 17 cooperative agreements funded for the CDC Smoke Alarm Installation and Fire-safety Education program. CDR Jackson is a commissioned officer in the U.S. Public Health Service and has more than 20 years of public health experience working in both the Indian Health Service and the CDC.

David E. Jacobs, PhD, CIH – Dr. Jacobs is research director at the National Center for Healthy Housing (NCHH) and an adjunct associate professor at the University of Illinois School of Public Health. Formerly Director of the Office of Healthy Homes and Lead Hazard Control at the U.S. Department of Housing and Urban Development, he is the principal author of a report to Congress that launched the nation's healthy housing initiative and a report for the President's Task Force regarding childhood lead poisoning prevention. He has published numerous studies on housing and health, holds degrees in environmental engineering, technology and science policy, environmental health (chemistry), and political science, and is a certified industrial hygienist.

Arnie Katz, MA Ed – Mr. Katz is director of training and senior building science consultant at Advanced Energy in Raleigh, North Carolina, where he has worked for 25 years. A former building contractor, Arnie was the founding director of Advanced Energy's Healthy Building Resource Center and is currently co-director of the North Carolina Healthy Homes Training Center, the NC affiliate of the NCHH. A member of NCHH's Technical Advisory Group, Arnie provides training for builders, trades contractors, code officials, architects, engineers, and designers across the country on techniques and technologies for building healthier, more durable, more comfortable, and more energy-efficient homes. He's a graduate of Duke University and his MA Ed is from Western Carolina University.

Karin A. Mack, PhD–Dr. Mack is a senior behavioral scientist in CDC's NCIPC. She is also an adjunct assistant professor in Emory University's Sociology Department. She has worked at CDC since 1997 and was previously an assistant professor of sociology at Mississippi State University. Dr. Mack also worked at the National Institute on Aging/National Institutes of Health (NIH) for 7 years. Dr. Mack's PhD. is from the University of Maryland, College Park, Maryland. Her BA is from James Madison College of Michigan State University. She has been a Section Councilor for the Injury Control and Emergency Health Services Section of the American Public Health Association (APHA) and is an APHA Publications Board member.

Angela Mickalide, PhD, CHES, is the director of education and outreach of the Home Safety Council. She is responsible for leading the development, execution, and evaluation of injury prevention outreach initiatives, educational campaigns, and community volunteer programs. For 15 years, Dr. Mickalide served as the program director of the National SAFE KIDS Campaign. Throughout her career, Dr. Mickalide has received numerous awards including the Early Career Award from APHA's Public Health Education and Health Promotion Section, a Health Service Commendation for exemplary performance as Staff Coordinator of the U.S. Preventive Services Task Force, and a Champion of SAFE KIDS Award. She also received the Sarah Mazelis Award for outstanding public health education practice from APHA Public Health Education and Health Promotion Section. Most recently, she was awarded the SOPHE Trophy by the organization's president for outstanding service as Trustee for Publications and Communications. She earned her PhD in 1985 at The Johns Hopkins University in Baltimore, Maryland. Dr. Mickalide is also a certified health education specialist.

Rebecca Morley, MSPP–Ms. Morley is the executive director of the National Center for Healthy Housing (NCHH). Ms. Morley led the development of the National Healthy Homes Training Center. Ms. Morley worked with the U.S. Department of Housing and Urban Development (HUD) in a variety of posts. She served on the President's Task Force for Children's Environmental Health Safety and contributed to HUD's preliminary Healthy Homes Initiative plan and Strategic Plan to Eliminate Childhood Lead Poisoning by 2010. She designed and implemented a national multimillion-dollar healthy homes education campaign focused on injury prevention. Ms. Morley also served as a legislative fellow to U.S. Senator Jack Reed, where she authored key components of the Kennedy Health Bill related to childhood lead poisoning and helped to establish a national childhood lead poisoning prevention week through a Senate resolution. Ms. Morley holds a bachelor's degree in environmental science and a master's degree in public policy from the Georgia Institute of Technology.

Daniel Morrison, BS–Mr. Morrison is managing editor at GreenBuildingAdvisor.com. He earned a degree in ecosystems biology from the University of Montana and headed off to the field to be a biologist. He hooted for spotted owls in Oregon and counted fish aboard a fishing trawler in the Bering Sea, Alaska. After realizing that spending five months at sea each year isn't conducive to having a family, he got a day job building houses. After ten years in residential construction, he answered a classified ad in his favorite magazine, *Fine Homebuilding*, for an assistant editor position, and a month later was sitting in a cubicle, learning to type. He was promoted to senior editor before being asked to help build a new green residential construction Web site with another publisher, BuildingGreen. He has a wife, two kids and a shaggy dog.

Mary Evelyn Northridge, PhD, MPH–Dr. Northridge is a professor of Clinical Sociomedical Sciences (in Dental Medicine) at Columbia University, and holds joint appointments in the Mailman School of Public Health (MSPH) and the College of Dental Medicine. Professor Northridge was reappointed editor-in-chief of the *American Journal of Public Health (AJPH)* for her fourth three-year term in July 2008, and has served as an editor of the *AJPH* since 1993. She earned a BA in chemistry with a specialty in biochemistry at the University of Virginia, an MPH in environmental health at the University of Medicine and Dentistry of New Jersey/Rutgers University, and a PhD in epidemiology at Columbia University. Professor Northridge continued her research and academic career at the Harlem Health Promotion Center of Columbia University, where she still serves as a co-investigator. She has enduring interests in social and environmental determinants of health, and the importance of safe and affordable housing to ensuring the public's health.

Jerome A. Paulson, MD, FAAP, is associate professor of pediatrics at the George Washington University School of Medicine and Health Sciences and associate professor of Prevention and Community Health and research associate professor of Environmental and Occupational Health at the George Washington School of Public Health and Health Services. He is medical director for National and Global Affairs of the Children's Health Advocacy Institute at the Children's National Medical Center. Dr. Paulson is one of the co-directors of the Mid-Atlantic Center for Children's Health and the Environment. He serves on the American Academy of Pediatrics Committee on Environmental Health and the Children's Health Protection Advisory Committee for the U.S. Environmental Protection Agency. In October 2004 he was a Dozor Visiting Professor at Ben Gurion University in Beer Sheva, Israel. He was a recipient of a Soros Advocacy Fellowship for Physicians from the Open Society Institute.

Joseph T. Ponessa, PhD–Dr. Ponessa recently retired from Rutgers Cooperative Extension after serving 25 years as the housing, indoor environment, and health specialist; he continues to be active in these areas. His work involves curriculum development and outreach education, primarily on the topics of the indoor environment and its impact on health; areas of special interest include radon issues, lead poisoning, asthma trigger management and mold issues. Related interests include management of building moisture problems and construction technology. He currently teaches one-day courses on building science for building code officials, and a new course on construction and indoor environmental quality. Dr. Ponessa serves as a consultant on several healthy homes projects and provides guest lectures on environmental and construction topics. His formal training is in medical physiology, and he has extensive experience in the building trades.

Megan Sandel, MD, MPH, FAAP–Dr. Sandel is an assistant professor of pediatrics at Boston University School of Medicine and is an attending physician in the Pediatric Environmental Health Specialty Unit for Region I. Her work has focused on asthma, lead, injuries, housing, and child health. Cited as a respected authority in her field, Dr. Sandel often gives testimony on the connection between housing and child health in the United States. She has served as a principal investigator on grants from HUD with the Boston Public Health Commission to study whether housing changes improved the health of children with asthma. She has a K award from NIH on housing and stress in urban children. In 2007, Dr Sandel was named medical director of the National Center for Medical Legal Partnership and serves on the Committee on Environmental Health at the American Academy of Pediatrics.

Fatemeh Shafiei, PhD–Dr. Shafiei is an associate professor of political science at Spelman College. She received her PhD from the University of California, Riverside, in 1990. Her research and teaching interests are in the areas of environmental policy, environmental justice, environmental education, and international relations. She has served as an environmental fellow at Associated Colleges of the South (2003–2008). Dr. Shafiei's work on environmental policy, particularly within the state of Georgia, resulted in her extensive analysis of environmental laws passed by the Georgia legislature, documented in nine chapters on environmental policy in the *Georgia Legislative Review*, an annual publication that analyzes broad public policy issues in the state. Dr. Shafiei has served as principal investigator on several grants from the U.S. Environmental Protection Agency (EPA). She also received a grant from the United Negro College Fund/Mellon Program for "Education for Sustainability: Greening the College Curriculum Institute." She was a Partnership Leader in the Education for Sustainability Project, a Department of Energy (DOE)–funded project.

Ellen R. Tohn, MCP–Ms. Tohn is an environmental and health consultant with more than 20 years of experience. She is the founder and principal of Tohn Environmental Strategies and a nationally recognized expert in housing-based environmental health threats, healthy housing and indoor air quality, and lead poisoning prevention. Ms. Tohn has assisted national, regional, and local health advocates in catalyzing effective and lasting policy solutions, contributed to numerous federal and state guidance documents; developed federal and local healthy housing and lead training courses, and designed and managed environmental health research studies. She recently directed a project to develop guidance for EPA's Energy Star Indoor Air Quality Specifications and serves as an advisor on indoor air quality issues to the U.S. Green Building Council's LEED for Homes standards-setting process and numerous other green building programs.

Charles (Chuck) D. Treser, MPH, DAAS—Mr. Treser is a senior lecturer in the Department of Environmental and Occupational Health Sciences, School of Public Health at the University of Washington in Seattle, Washington. In 1971, he began his career in environmental health as an environmental health inspector with the Allegheny County Health Department in Pittsburgh, Pennsylvania, working primarily in the housing and community environment programs. In 1976, Mr. Treser received his MPH degree from the University of Michigan. In 1980 he moved to the University of Washington, where he teaches both undergraduate and graduate students. He is an active participant in the University of Washington's Northwest Center for Public Health Practice, through which he manages a partnership with the NCHH to teach healthy housing courses in the Northwest. His awards include the Washington State Public Health Association's Tom Drummey Award and the APHA Environment Section's Distinguished Service Award. Mr. Treser was the first president of the Association of Environmental Health Academic Programs (AEHAP) and is the principal investigator on a cooperative agreement between AEHAP and CDC. Mr. Treser also served as the chair of the International EH Faculty Forum from 2002 to 2004.

Lynn Underwood, BA, BS, is a Building Official with the city of Norfolk, Virginia. He has worked in the building safety profession and building code development for 26 years and has held additional positions such as inspector, property maintenance inspector, combination inspector, plan reviewer, senior plans examiner, assistant building official and building code official. He is fully certified in all aspects of construction by the International Code Council (ICC) and sits on three national code development committees. He is immediate past president and board member with the Virginia Building and Code Official's Association. He led a team of inspectors to El Salvador on behalf of the CASA Corps (ICC Ad Hoc Group) to inspect restoration work performed by USAID projects. This trip and previous committee work also served as an outreach to areas of Latin America for ICC and led, in part, to the translation of the I Codes into Spanish. Before college, Lynn enlisted in the USMC and served in Vietnam with the 1st Marine Division. He was awarded several medals including a Purple Heart and Navy Commendation, and a Meritorious Combat promotion.

Joseph L. Wysocki, PhD—Dr. Wysocki, with more than 40 years of teaching and research experience, has been the National Program Leader for Housing and Indoor Environments, The National Institute of Food and Agriculture, U.S. Department of Agriculture since 1991. Previously, Dr. Wysocki was a professor and extension housing specialist for 14 years with the University of Illinois and The Pennsylvania State University. His doctorate degree, in consumer economics and housing, is from Cornell University. As National Program Leader, he provides national direction for research, education, and extension/outreach programs on sustainable and healthy housing issues including economics, energy, environmental health and safety, and disaster education. In 1988, Dr. Wysocki was the first recipient of the Distinguished Service Award from the Housing Education and Research Association.

Introduction: A Systems Science Approach to Promoting Healthy Homes

Mary E. Northridge, PhD, MPH, and
Annie Feighery, MPA, EdM

> *There is something in all of us that loves to put together a puzzle,*
> *that loves to see the image of the whole emerge. The beauty of a*
> *person, or a flower, or a poem lies in seeing all of it. It is interest-*
> *ing that the words "whole" and "health" come from the same root*
> *(the Old English* hal, *as in "hale" and "hearty"). So it should come*
> *as no surprise that the unhealthiness of our world today is in direct*
> *proportion to our inability to see it as a whole. (Senge 2006, p. 68)*

It is both a sobering and an opportune time for the writing and publication of this volume devoted to healthy homes. The U.S. foreclosure activity in April 2009 jumped 32% from a year earlier to a record high; 1 of every 374 U.S. households with mortgages received a foreclosure filing in that month alone (Adler 2009). On June 9, 2009, the U.S. Surgeon General released a *Call to Action to Promote Healthy Homes*, which underscores the public health import of housing and housing interventions (U.S. Department of Health and Human Services 2009). This report opens with a broad vision of what is meant by the term "healthy home," that is, "A healthy home is sited, designed, built, renovated, and maintained in ways that support the health of residents" (U.S. Department of Health and Human Services 2009).

The field of public health was born out of the squalid conditions of the industrialized cities of the nineteenth century; the improvement of housing and neighborhoods has always been a core activity of the field and a central component of tackling poverty (Chadwick 1943; Engels 1892; Riis 1890). However, scientific contributions to enhancing healthy homes have tended to be episodic, underfunded, overly narrow, and in need of a comprehensive, purposeful, sustained vision. In this chapter, the evidence base for the connections between housing and health will be examined, with an emphasis on comprehensive reviews that were published in the peer-reviewed literature. Second, useful frameworks that can inform relevant policy and action to promote healthy homes will be highlighted, with a focus on systems science as an adaptive, dynamic, evolutionary, and yet pragmatic approach that holds promise for future advances. Third, selected examples of successful housing interventions will be discussed, especially those that focus on vulnerable populations, such as children, older adults, and historically oppressed and disadvantaged subgroups. Finally, the importance of metaphor as an integrative tool will be explained (Pickett, Cadenasso, and Grove 2004) and endorsed as a way of linking public health with other vital fields to create a more holistic, systems science approach to promoting and sustaining healthy homes, healthy neighborhoods, and healthy societies.

REVIEWING THE EVIDENCE

Howden-Chapman (2004) designed an accessible and thoughtfully organized glossary of housing and health that accounts for diverse disciplinary and policy traditions, and identifies the aspects of housing that can provide a basis for concerted research and action. She believes that houses and neighborhoods are very practical settings for public health action, and by their nature, combine both private and public interests. Nonetheless, she concluded that current interventions are limited by their scope and narrow definitions of housing and health (Howden-Chapman 2004).

Scientific articles on housing and health research are framed by a few seminal reviews that are frequently cited. Feinstein (1993) realized the complexity of the relationship between socioeconomic status and health, and sought to organize the various explanations for health inequalities along two dimensions. He identified two major sources of inequality: (1) disparities arising from different experiences over the life span (diet, smoking, exercise, and occupation) and (2) access to and use of the formal health care system. He also recognized two types of explanations: (1) behavioral (psychological, genetic, and cultural) and (2) materialistic (wealth, home ownership, automobile ownership). Under materialistic lifestyle effects, he explicitly included housing, overcrowding, sanitation, transit mode, occupational hazards, and environmental hazards. He was prescient in calling for investment in interdisciplinary modeling that might ultimately use computer simulation techniques to map out life span risk and mortality portfolios (Feinstein 1993).

Shaw (2004) argued convincingly for a long-term view of housing and health. Although public health maintains a historic link with the improvement of housing, Shaw believes that too much attention has been focused on individualistic lifestyle factors in recent decades, rather than on issues of socioeconomic structure. As income distribution has become more unequal, the matter of housing affordability has become more pressing for an increasing number of people throughout the world. Shaw (2004) concluded that investment in housing can be more than an investment in bricks and mortar—it can also form a foundation for the health and well-being of populations. She developed a heuristic device to comprehensively consider the direct and indirect ways in which housing can affect health. Figure 1.1 shows an adaptation of this device based on features of the built environment and social context (Schulz and Northridge 2004).

According to Dunn (2000), there is a growing awareness that one of the most important research needs in health inequalities scholarship is to better elucidate those pathways by which differences in socioeconomic status manifest in everyday life and produce, at the aggregate level, the systematic social gradient in health observed in all industrialized countries. His review of the literature on housing and health found little empirical work that explicitly investigated housing as a factor in the social production of health inequalities. A later empirical investigation by Dunn (2002) among Vancouver residents found support for the hypothesis that

	Direct		Indirect
	Individual/household level		*Community/neighborhood level*
Built environment	Material/physical effects of housing on health (damp, mold, cold, heat)	Income and wealth to afford housing	Availability of services, facilities, transportation systems
		Proximity to services, facilities, transportation systems	
Social context	Financial insecurity, debt, foreclosure	Household and community cultures and health behaviors	
	Feeling of "home," social status, well-being		Civic participation and social integration

Source: Adapted from Shaw, M. Housing and Public Health. Annu Rev of Public Health. (2004) 25: 397-418 based on Schulz, A., and M.E. Northridge. Social determinants of health: Implications for environmental health promotion. Health Educ Behav (2004):31:455–71.

Figure 1.1 — Direct and indirect (built environment and social context) pathways by which housing can affect health.

features of the domestic environment, especially as they pertain to the exercise of control and the experience of demand, are significant predictors of self-reported general and mental health status. In his view, housing is a concrete manifestation of socioeconomic status, which has an important role to play in the development of explanations of the social production of health inequalities (Dunn 2002).

Pickett and Pearl (2001) were interested in the effects of neighborhood or local-area socioeconomic characteristics on health (see also Kawachi and Berkman 2000), and thus conducted a systematic review of the evidence on this subtopic. Notwithstanding the heterogeneity in designs and methods, substitution of local-area measures for neighborhood measures, and probable measurement error, Pickett and Pearl found that modest neighborhood effects on health were fairly consistently demonstrated across studies. They also succeeded in drawing public health attention to the health risks associated with the social structure and ecology of neighborhoods, with the hope that innovative approaches to community interventions might ensue (Pickett and Pearl 2001). In another widely cited article, Krieger and Higgins (2002) reviewed a range of health conditions associated with poor housing conditions, including infectious diseases, chronic illnesses, injuries, poor nutrition, and mental disorders. They compared the housing interventions used by health officials in the nineteenth century—which targeted poor sanitation, crowding, and inadequate ventilation to reduce infectious diseases, as well as fire hazards to decrease injuries—with the multiple housing strategies available to public health departments today, namely, developing and enforcing housing guidelines and codes, implementing "Healthy Homes" programs to improve indoor air quality, assessing housing conditions, and advocating for healthy, affordable housing (Krieger and Higgins 2002).

Lawrence (2006) contrasted traditional disciplinary studies, which are sector-based, with interdisciplinary contributions that offer a broader approach. In particular, he cited the biomedical model that often adopts a symptom–treatment interpretation of housing and health as being narrowly focused when contrasted with holistic, integrated models that combine biological, cultural, economic, political, psychological, and social factors in new ways.

Beyond these foundational reviews on housing and health are several outstanding analyses that examine housing intervention studies per se. Thomson, Petticrew, and Morrison (2001) conducted a systematic review of experimental and non experimental housing intervention studies that measured quantitative health outcomes dating from 1887. Only 18 completed primary intervention studies were identified; 11 were prospective, 6 of which included control groups. The authors attributed the lack of evidence linking housing and health to pragmatic difficulties with housing studies and unfavorable political climates, and called for large-scale studies that investigate the wider social context of housing interventions (Thomson, Petticrew, and Morrison 2001).

Eight years later, Thomson et al. (2009) conducted a more comprehensive, systemic review of the health impacts of housing improvement. Forty-two bibliographic databases were searched for housing interventions from 1887 to 2007, and 45 relevant studies were identified. Those from the developing world suggested that the provision of basic housing amenities may lead to reduced illness. Overall, Thomson et al. (2009) concluded that warmth improvements in particular can lead to tangible improvements in health, but the potential may depend on baseline housing conditions and careful targeting of the intervention.

Saegert et al. (2003) conducted a content analysis of 72 articles selected from 12 electronic databases of U.S. public health interventions related to housing published from 1990 to 2001. The overwhelming majority (92%) of interventions addressed a single condition, most often lead poisoning, asthma, or injury, and approximately half (52%) targeted children. The salient qualities of the most successful interventions were that they (1) were policy based and relatively cost effective; (2) targeted technological improvements that were effective, cheap, and durable; and (3) involved affected people more deeply in the solutions, especially through home visits. They ended with a call for more ecologically grounded interventions, which is one of the conceptual frameworks described next.

FRAMING THE ISSUES

In this section, we have chosen to be selective by design to cogently explain three conceptual frameworks that have proven fruitful in advancing research and action on healthy homes, healthy neighborhoods, and healthy societies. Although the frameworks are known by various model titles in the scientific literature, we have elected to refer to them as the following core yet inclusive and unifying terms: ecological models, health impact assessment (HIA), and systems science.

Northridge, Sclar, and Biswas (2003) presented an ecological model for navigating pathways and planning healthy cities that is centrally concerned with the social, political, economic, and historical processes that generate the urban built environment. The authors posit that three domains—the natural environment (including topography, climate, and water supply), macrosocial factors (including historical conditions, political and economic orders, and human rights doctrines), and inequalities (including those related to the distribution of wealth, employment and educational opportunities, and political influence)—contain the fundamental factors that underlie and influence health and well-being via multiple pathways through differential access to power, information, and resources (Link and Phelan 1995). Fundamental factors, in turn, influence two broad domains of intermediate factors: the built environment (including land use, transportations systems, and buildings) and the social context (including community investment, public and fiscal policies, and civic participation). Next, the proximate factors consist of two major domains: stressors (including violent crime, financial insecurity, and environmental toxins) and social integration and social support (including the shape of networks and the resources available within networks). Finally, health is conceived as consisting of two interconnected domains: health outcomes (e.g., obesity, injury and violence, and respiratory health) and well-being (e.g., hope/despair, life satisfaction, and happiness).

A second important approach toward promoting healthy homes is HIA, which is commonly defined as a combination of procedures, methods, and tools by which a policy, program, or project may be judged in terms of its potential effects on the health of a population, and the distribution of those effects within the population (Dannenberg et al. 2006). HIA has been endorsed by certain health agencies because of increased awareness that community design, land use, transportation systems, and other environmental and social factors affect the health of populations, even as the health sector often lacks requisite expertise in other relevant sectors. According to Dannenberg et al. (2006), the conduct of an HIA includes the following five steps: (1) *screening* to identify projects or policies for which an HIA would be useful; (2) *scoping* to identify which health impacts should be assessed and which populations are affected; (3) *assessing* the magnitude, direction, and certainty of health impacts; (4) *reporting* the results to decision makers; and (5) *evaluating* the effect of the HIA on the decision-making process. Although HIA has the potential to enhance recognition of societal determinants of health and responsibility for health across sectors (e.g., public health, urban planning, environmental protection), greater clarity is required regarding criteria for initiating, conducting, and completing HIA, including rules pertaining to decision making, enforcement, compliance, and paying for their conduct (Krieger et al. 2003).

Finally, Leischow and Milstein (2006) define a systems science approach that holds great potential for advancing healthy homes as a paradigm or perspective that considers connections among different components (e.g., stocks and flows of afflicted people, adverse housing conditions, resources for community health protection), plans for the implications of their interaction, and requires interdisciplinary thinking and active engagement of those who have a stake in the outcome to govern the course of change. Figure 1.2 presents a system dynamics–type diagram for thinking about the dynamics of housing and health in these broader terms.

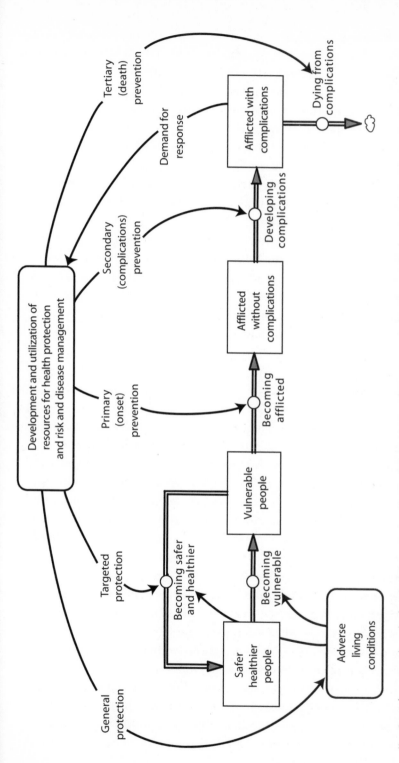

Note. Rectangles represent the stocks of people; thick arrows with circles represent flows of people; thinner arrows indicate causal influence; rounded rectangles indicate multidimensional concepts. With permission from Homer, J.P., and G.B. Hirsch. System dynamics modeling for public health: Background and opportunities. Am J Public Health (2006):96:452–8.

Figure 1.2 — A broad view of housing and health and the spectrum of possible responses.

Figure 1.2 moves beyond diagramming to explore a more complete view of health by means of simulation. This community health model examines the typical feedback interactions among broadly defined states of affliction prevalence, adverse housing conditions, and the capacity of the community to act. Sensitivity testing of the model across many possible community and affliction characteristics is intended to lead to conclusions about how different types of outside assistance are likely to affect a community in the short and long term (Homer and Hirsch 2006).

Although systems science has much intuitive appeal, it is also increasingly endorsed by authoritative U.S. public health bodies—including the Institute of Medicine (Plsek 2001), the National Institutes of Health (Mabry et al. 2008), and the Centers for Disease Control and Prevention (Gerberding 2005)—as an approach that merits further development. Midgley (2006) offers a methodology for systemic intervention that 1) emphasizes the need to explore stakeholder values and boundaries, 2) challenges marginalization, and 3) draws upon a wide range of methods to create a flexible and responsive systems science practice. Case studies from the scientific literature that use each of these conceptual models toward improving housing and health are detailed in the following section.

INTERVENING SUCCESSFULLY

In this section, we focus on case studies of housing interventions that were targeted to assist vulnerable subpopulations who are disproportionately burdened with poor housing and are more susceptible to experiencing poor health because of environmental hazards when compared with the general population. Spielman et al. (2006) used an ecological model for addressing childhood asthma as part of the Harlem Children's Zone Asthma Initiative. Given the emphasis on children with asthma and their built environment (notably housing and schools), the investigators modified the model presented by Northridge, Sclar, and Biswas (2003) to examine relationships among racial, ethnic, and social inequalities at the societal level; the built environment and social context at the community level; stressors and buffers at the interpersonal level; and disparities in health and well-being among individuals and across populations (see Figure 2 in Spielman et al. 2006).

They found that aspects of home environments within the control of the parents and guardians of children with asthma improved significantly over the course of the program, including statistically significant reductions in dust, mold, spray bombs, incense, smoking in the home, and perfume (Spielman et al. 2006). However, no important changes were found in reported problems with mice or cockroaches during the first year. Although this project provided environmental education and integrated pest management services to families who reported problems with mice and cockroaches, these findings suggest that pest management at the scale of the individual household is not effective in multifamily buildings such as those in Central Harlem, New York City.

Bhatia (2007) provided a detailed account of two instances in which the San Francisco Department of Public Health used a form of HIA to account for societal-level health determinants that are not traditionally evaluated in land-use decisions. The first case study concerned the demolition of Trinity Plaza Apartments (360 rent-controlled units) and the construction of 1400 condominiums. Residents and tenant advocates challenged the determination of no adverse housing impacts by the Department of City Planning, arguing that displacement of people would lead to mental stress and the destruction of a cohesive community. A review by the San Francisco Department of Public Health subsequently identified several health consequences of the redevelopment proposal: psychological stress, fear, and insecurity caused by eviction; crowded or substandard living conditions because of limited affordable replacement housing; food insecurity or hunger caused by increased rent burdens; and loss of supportive social networks owing to displacement.

As a result of the HIA, the Department of City Planning revised its determination for the Trinity Plaza proposal accordingly. The developer ultimately agreed to negotiate with the tenants, and a revised proposal called for the replacement of the 360 rent-controlled units, continued leases for the existing tenants, a 1000-square-foot meeting space, and a children's play structure (Bhatia 2006).

A final illustrative case study is provided by Midgley (2006), who stresses critical examination of values, boundaries, and marginalization in his systems science approach to public health intervention. Briefly, the project involved working with local governments in the United Kingdom to determine how information from assessments of older adults applying for health, housing, and welfare services could be aggregated to inform the development of housing policy. Two major problems quickly became manifest. First, if the housing "needs" expressed by older adults fell outside of local government spending priorities, they were not recorded. Second, many urgent problems with service provision, assessment, and multi-agency planning were raised; to ignore them would be unethical. Thus, the study was expanded to instead examine the larger system of assessment, information provision, and multi-agency planning for housing for older adults and what could be done to improve it.

Midgley (2006) used this case study to demonstrate the benefits of boundary critique: the initial project proposal was usefully expanded, and the potential for marginalizing older adults was identified and addressed. In addition, a combination of semistructured interviewing, problem mapping, interactive planning, critical systems heuristics, and viable system modeling was used over the course of this intervention. In Midgley's view, no single set of methods yet developed could have addressed all of the relevant issues that were involved. Instead, "methodological pluralism" supported the stakeholders in both defining the issue and responding to it systematically (Midgley 2006).

LINKING HOUSING AND HEALTH

We close this chapter with a contribution by Pickett (1999), who proposed metaphor as a powerful tool for creating new ideas and syntheses, and suggested how to use an idea or approach developed in one realm in an entirely different realm. This idea resonated with us as we wrestled with how to integrate the various sectors necessary to bring about improved population health through safe and affordable housing. Is "healthy homes" a sufficiently powerful metaphor for this purpose?

Pickett, Cadenasso, and Grove (2004) critically examined the metaphor of "cities of resilience" for its ability to promote closer linkage among the disciplines of urban design, ecology, and social science. They also pointed to earlier uses of metaphor in planning, including "The City Beautiful," which focused on the aesthetics of grand buildings and their landscaped settings, and "The Garden City," in which large productive and recreational green spaces were zoned as an isolated counterpoise to crowded commercial, residential, and industrial sectors (Pickett, Cadenasso, and Grove 2004).

Approximately two decades ago, Sclar (1990) denounced homelessness and housing policy by likening the dynamic linkage between the structural loss of housing resources and the personal loss of shelter to the children's game of "musical chairs." Sclar used this metaphor because he believed it was essential for public health professionals to give special prominence to explaining the linkage between the structural factors that create the potential for a high prevalence of homelessness and the personal factors that determine who are most susceptible.

Over the past year, the U.S. federal government has devoted substantial resources to shore up financial markets, yet the number of housing foreclosures in 2009 is expected to outpace the record number of housing foreclosures in 2008 by one third. In response, U.S. Senator Jack Reed (D-RI) has introduced legislation known as the Preserving Homes and Communities Act of 2009, which is intended to address the housing crisis by requiring that qualified homeowners are evaluated for and offered loan modifications, establishing a new mortgage payment assistance program, and providing incentives to states and local governments to create strong mediation programs (see http://reed.senate.gov/newsroom/details.cfm?id=318453).

The past year has also highlighted the possibility for systems science to enable us to better understand and address complex, dynamic, interconnected issues, as embodied in a proposed "healthy homes" approach. The approach encourages the integration of fields that typically operate in isolation, for example, public health, urban planning, pest management, air quality, hazard abatement, water quality, and heating and cooling systems. We believe "healthy homes" will be powerful as a metaphor to bring about essential research and action to the extent that it allows us to see this societal priority more broadly and holistically. Although we are hopeful about the potential of a systems science approach to better achieve healthy homes, healthy neighborhoods, and healthy societies, we endorse a plurality of theories, methods, and tools to solve this historically intransient social ill. In the words of Meadows (2008, p. 6–7):

> At a time when the world is more messy, more crowded, more interconnected, more interdependent, and more rapidly changing than ever before, the more ways of seeing, the better. The systems-thinking lens allows us to reclaim our intuition about whole systems and hone our abilities to understand parts, see interconnections, ask 'what-if' questions about possible future behaviors, and be creative and courageous about system redesign. Then we can use our insights to make a difference in ourselves and our world.

ACKNOWLEDGMENTS
Dr. Northridge and Ms. Feighery were supported in the conceptualization, research, and writing of this chapter by contract 7–78438 from the American Legacy Foundation (Principal Investigator: Northridge) and development grant 4–25917 from the Department of Sociomedical Sciences, Columbia University Mailman School of Public Health (Principal Investigator: Northridge).

REFERENCES
Adler, L. *U.S. Foreclosures Jump to Record High.* New York, NY: Reuters, 2009. Available at: http://www.reuters.com/article/newsOne/idUSTRE54C0OR20090513.

Bhatia, R. Protecting health using an Environmental Impact Assessment: A case study of San Francisco land use decision making. *Am J Public Health* (2007):97:406–13.

Chadwick, E. *Report on the Sanitary Condition of the Labouring Population of Great Britain.* London, UK: W. Clowes and Sons, 1943 (original published 1842).

Dannenberg, A.L., R. Bhatia, B.L. Cole, et al. Growing the field of health impact assessment in the United States: An agenda for research and practice. *Am J Public Health* (2006):96:262–70.

Dunn, J.R. Housing and health inequalities: Review and prospects for research. *Housing Studies* (2000):15:341–66.

——. Housing and inequalities in health: A study of socioeconomic dimensions of housing and self reported health from a survey of Vancouver residents. *J Epidemiol Community Health* (2002):56:671–81.

Engels, F. *The Condition of the Working Class in England in 1844.* London, U.K.: Swan Sonnenschein & Co., 1892. Note: Originally published in German in 1845 by Leipzig under the title *Die Lage der arbeitenden Klasse in England.*

Feinstein, J.S. The relationship between socioeconomic status and health: A review of the literature. *Milbank Q* (1993):71:279–322.

Gerberding, J.L. Protecting health—the new research imperative. *JAMA* (2005):294:1403–6.

Homer, J.P., and G.B. Hirsch. System dynamics modeling for public health: Background and opportunities. *Am J Public Health* (2006):96:452–8.

Howden-Chapman, P. Housing standards: A glossary of housing and health. *J Epidemiol Community Health* (2004):58:162–8.

Kawachi, I., and L.F. Berkman, eds. *Neighborhoods and Health.* New York, NY: Oxford University Press, Inc., 2000.

Krieger, J., and D.L. Higgins. Housing and health: Time again for public health action. *Am J Public Health* (2002):92:758–68.

Krieger, N., M. Northridge, S. Gruskin, et al. Assessing health impact assessment: Multidisciplinary and international perspectives. *J Epidemiol Community Health* (2003):57:659–62.

Lawrence, R.J. Housing and health: Beyond disciplinary confinement. *J Urban Health* (2006):83:540–9.

Leischow, S.J., and B. Milstein. Systems thinking and modeling for public health practice. *Am J Public Health* (2006):96:403–5.

Link, B.G., and J. Phelan. Social conditions as fundamental causes of disease. *J Health Soc Behav* (1995):Spec. No.:80–94. Review.

Mabry, P.L., D.H. Olster, G.D. Morgan, and D.B. Abrams. Interdisciplinary and systems science to improve population health: A view from the NIH Office of Behavioral and Social Sciences Research. *Am J Prev Med* (2008):35:211–24.

Meadows, D.H. *Thinking in Systems: A Primer.* White River Junction, VT: Chelsea Green Publishing, 2008.

Midgley, G. Systemic intervention for public health. *Am J Public Health* (2006):96:466–72.

Northridge, M.E., E. Sclar, and P. Biswas. Sorting out the connections between the built environment and health: A conceptual framework for navigating pathways and planning healthy cities. *J Urban Health* (2003):80:556–68.

Pickett, S.T.A. The culture of synthesis: Habits of mind in novel ecological integration. *Oikos* (1999):87:479–87.

Pickett, S.T.A., M.L. Cadenasso, and J.M. Grove. Resilient cities: Meaning, models, and metaphor for integrating the ecological, socio-economic, and planning realms. *Landsc Urban Plan* (2004):69:369–84.

Pickett, K.E., and M. Pearl. Multilevel analyses of neighbourhood socioeconomic context and health outcomes: A critical review. *J Epidemiol Community Health* (2001):55:111–22.

Plsek, P. Appendix B: Redesigning health care with insights from the science of complex adaptive systems. In: Committee on Quality of Health Care in America, editor. *Crossing the Quality Chasm: A New Health System for the 21st Century*. Washington, DC: Institute of Medicine, 2001:309–322.

Riis, J. *How the Other Half Lives: Studies Among the Tenements of New York*. New York, NY: Charles Scribner's Sons, 1890.

Saegert, S.C., S. Klitzman, N. Freudenberg, J. Cooperman-Mroczek, and S. Nassar. Healthy housing: A structured review of published evaluations of U.S. interventions to improve health by modifying housing in the United States, 1990–2001. *Am J Public Health* (2003):93:1471–7.

Schulz, A, and M.E. Northridge. Social determinants of health: Implications for environmental health promotion. *Health Educ Behav* (2004):31:455–71.

Sclar, E. Homelessness and housing policy: A game of musical chairs. *Am J Public Health* (1990):80:1039–40.

Senge, P.M. *The Fifth Discipline: The Art & Practice of the Learning Organization*. New York, NY: Doubleday, 2006.

Shaw, M. Housing and public health. *Annu Rev Public Health* (2004):25:397–418.

Spielman, S.E., C.A. Golembeski, M.E. Northridge, et al. Interdisciplinary planning for healthier communities: Findings from the Harlem Children's Zone Asthma Initiative. *J Am Plann Assoc* (2006):72:100–8.

Thomson, H., M. Petticrew, and D. Morrison. Health effects of housing improvement: Systematic review of intervention studies. *BMJ* (2001):323:187–90.

Thomson, H., S. Thomas, E. Sellstrom, and M. Petticrew. The health impacts of housing improvement: A systematic review of intervention studies from 1887 to 2007. *Am J Public Health* 2009:99(Suppl 3):S681–92. Review.

U.S. Department of Health and Human Services. *The Surgeon General's Call to Action to Promote Healthy Homes*. Washington, DC: U.S. Department of Health and Human Services, Office of the Surgeon General, 2009. Available at: http://www.surgeongeneral.gov/topics/healthyhomes/calltoactiontopromotehealthyhomes.pdf. Accessed August 9, 2010.

Principles of Healthy Housing: Dry, Ventilated, Contaminant-Free, Pest-Free, Clean, Maintained

David Jacobs, PhD, and Jerry Hershovitz, BA

Housing conditions can and should support good health. This simple principle lies at the heart of the many interactions among certain housing characteristics and disease, injury, and overall well-being. Properly identifying those characteristics is a prerequisite to correcting housing conditions before they produce harm. Frameworks that organize the varied housing and health connections are reviewed in Chapters 1 and 4, but in general they are typically organized by multiple housing and community factors that are either proximate or distal to health. Examples of a proximate factor include a broken stair, which can lead to a fall, and deteriorated lead paint, which can lead to lead poisoning. A more distal factor includes inadequate job opportunities, which in turn promote inadequate housing investment, leading to deferred maintenance and the appearance of housing health hazards over time.

These efforts to group housing characteristics that matter to health are important, because they influence how we assess healthy housing and identify factors as housing hazards. In this chapter, we expand the traditional view that housing deficiencies are violations of specialized local housing codes, for example, plumbing, fire, mechanical, electrical, or other specific problems. Although such codes are important, they often do not address those housing factors associated with the chronic, more subtle forms of disease and injury, such as asthma, mold-induced illness, lead poisoning, and falls, which have emerged as new public health threats in recent years. This chapter shows how the specialized, segmented, categoric approach can be augmented by a more holistic approach to produce a more rational method of solving housing deficiencies that compromise health.

In 1946 the World Health Organization adopted an affirmative definition of health as a state of well-being beyond simply the lack of disease or infirmity. The definition states, "Health is a state of complete physical, mental and social well-being and not merely the absence of disease or infirmity." Therefore, to be healthy, a house must go beyond limiting or eliminating injury, disability, or disease as a result of interactions between a structure and its residents; a healthy home *supports* healthy behavior by residents. To fully implement this broader definition of health as it applies to housing, the categoric specialized code inspector model must be augmented by a more holistic approach. In addition, the definition of housing must be expanded beyond a single structure or building to include the grounds (premises), outbuildings, and the neighborhood, as well as its design, location, construction, repair, and renovation. Thus, healthy houses are dwellings and premises that are built, maintained, and repaired in a manner conducive to good occupant health and linked to social networks and healthy neighborhoods. Methods of assessing healthy housing must consider these other surrounding and supportive factors as well as the structure itself.

THE SUCCESS OF CHILDHOOD LEAD POISONING PREVENTION— IMPLICATIONS FOR OTHER HOUSING-RELATED DISEASES

When policies have been based on good scientific research, the substantial benefits of making healthy homes investments have become known and great progress has been possible, as is the case with childhood lead poisoning prevention from exposure to residential lead-based paint hazards.

Exposure to lead, a potent neurotoxicant, remains one of the most important and best studied household environmental risks to children (Agency for Toxic Substances and Disease Registry 2007; National Research Council 1993). Even so-called low levels of exposure have been associated with a host of behavioral, neurologic, and developmental adverse effects (Levin et al. 2008). Measures to eliminate or reduce the use of lead in a range of products—including gasoline, food and beverage cans, new residential paint, and potable water conduits—contributed to a dramatic decline in blood lead levels in all population groups from the mid-1970s to 2006 (Levin et al. 2008). In the late 1980s, 1.7 million U.S. preschoolers still had blood lead levels in a range in which subtle adverse effects on neurodevelopment have been established, but more recent data show that this number has declined to approximately 250,000, suggesting that further action is needed (Jones et al. 2009). A large reservoir of lead remains in housing built before the leaded paint ban in 1978 (Consumer Product Safety Commission 1977), especially in homes constructed before 1950, when white lead paint pigment was still widely used. The most recent published national survey from the U.S. Department of Housing and Urban Development (HUD) shows that 24 million units have lead-based paint hazards in the form of deteriorated lead-based paint and contaminated dust and soil (Jacobs et al. 2002). Strategies that include proper identification of lead paint hazards and contaminated dust and soil permit targeted lead hazard control work to proceed where it will have the greatest benefit. Typical hazard control actions include stabilizing deteriorated leaded paint, replacing windows or treating windows to reduce abrasion of leaded paint, covering bare contaminated soil, installing an enclosure, sealing floor surfaces, and performing specialized cleaning and clearance (dust) testing. Depending on the specific house, it may be advisable to remove all lead paint. Numerous studies have shown that modern lead hazard control is effective (National Center for Healthy Housing 2004; U.S. Environmental Protection Agency [EPA] 1998; Wilson et al. 2006). Other studies have also shown that if proper environmental controls are not in place during the work, exposure can actually increase, not decrease (Ashengrau et al. 1997; Farfel and Chisolm 1990; Farfel, Chisolm, and Rohde 1994; HUD 1995). If lead hazard control is done properly, the monetary benefits are enormous. Recent estimates of controlling lead-based paint hazards in housing are $67 billion in net benefits, including increased intelligence quotient (and thus increased productivity and lifetime earnings), increased market value, and improved energy efficiency (Nevin et al. 2008).

The lead experience holds important lessons for examining other housing-based environmental health hazards. Other sources of lead, such as lead in air, water, and food canning, can be controlled by addressing point sources, water chemistry, or a few manufacturing processes, respectively. On the other hand, lead-based paint hazards in housing constitute a decentralized yet highly concentrated exposure source, much like other housing-related health hazards.

Initial responses to the problem focused on simplistic, and in some cases harmful, removal of lead paint, as the distinction between lead-based paint and the conditions that made it a hazard were not well understood. Scientific research helped to uncover the previously unrecognized pathway of exposure from lead paint to settled lead house dust to contamination of children's hands, ingestion of lead through hand-to-mouth contact, and subsequent elevation of children's blood lead levels (Bornschein et al. 1987). This scientific finding fueled new housing and public health policy that focused on prevention of exposure and not simplistic removal of lead paint (Title X 1992). The policy also resulted in the creation of health-based residential lead exposure limits; a licensed and trained nationwide work force; laboratory quality-control, quality-assurance programs; occupational exposure standards for construction workers; and disclosure of known lead-based paint hazards at the time of sale or rental. In addition, the policy also resulted in public assistance for those homeowners who are not able to afford lead hazard control. All of these advances have profound implications for the tasks confronting the emerging healthy housing field.

The following sections trace the history of housing and health as well as the key housing factors that should be examined and remediated to produce a healthy home.

HOUSING LAWS AND HEALTH — THE BEGINNINGS

The first housing laws were developed to protect and promote health. A more complete accounting is available in the *Healthy Housing Reference Manual* (Centers for Disease Control and Prevention [CDC] and HUD 2006), which traces how the evolution of human society affected its housing, from the most primitive structures associated with hunter/gatherers that merely provided some protection against weather and the elements to the more complex buildings today that promote physical and mental health, comfort, and social well-being. Many modern housing and building codes trace their ancestry to the response to infectious disease epidemics that occurred with rapid industrialization and urbanization in Western countries more than 100 years ago. There is little doubt that improvements in housing in the developed countries have greatly advanced public health since then. Early housing standards required improved ventilation, sanitation, reduced crowding, structural soundness, lighting, and other habitability criteria, in part as a response to the appearance of concentrated slum housing around factories and big cities during the industrial revolution (Riis 1890).

The public health and housing movements have common roots in the efforts to clean up squalid conditions in slum housing a century ago. For example, indoor plumbing, still lacking in much of the developing world, helped improve sanitation and the control of cholera and other similar diseases in the developed world. Inadequate ventilation and crowding in housing contributed to the tuberculosis epidemic a century ago in the United States (Stein 1950) and remains a significant problem in developing countries today. The lack of indoor plumbing and basic sanitation was not initially recognized as a housing deficiency at first, because housing was initially intended to provide protection against the elements, little more. These housing changes made a powerful contribution to conquering these epidemics. Furthermore, improved sanitation through indoor plumbing, the creation of cleanable interior surfaces, better food preservation, and storage facilities in housing were clearly linked to other key advances in public health. Despite these rich historical examples, inadequate housing remains a major worldwide problem (World Health Organization 2005).

The Tenement House Act of 1901 attempted to reduce disease and so-called moral disintegration among impoverished immigrants on the lower east side of New York City by requiring improved light, ventilation, and indoor toilet facilities (Dolkart n.d.). Despite this early interest in the relationship between household crowding and disease, adverse health effects as a result of crowding continue to be documented. For example, the Housing, Crowding and Health Study conducted in New Zealand in 2003–2004 found that meningococcal disease in children was 4–5 times more prevalent in children in the most crowded quintile of neighborhoods (Baker et al. 2000). Poor housing conditions are known to be associated with mental and physical health risks. A study of New York City neighborhoods found that living in neighborhoods with poorer-quality housing is associated with an increased likelihood of depression (Galea, Freudenberg, and Vlahov 2005). The physical effects of the increased stress of living in substandard housing have been studied (Evans, Wells, and Moch 2003). A cumulative environmental risk of noise, crowding, and housing quality was positively correlated with elevated levels of overnight epinephrine, norepinephrine, and cortisol in a low-income sample group, but not in the middle-income group.

This historical experience demonstrates that the most effective way to address housing conditions leading to poor health is a multifactorial, multidisciplinary, holistic method, not a segmented, categoric approach. The publication of the *Basic Housing Inspection Manual* (U.S. Public Health Service 1975) by the American Public Health Association and the CDC helped to ensure that health considerations remained at the core of housing requirements. Yet in intervening years, categoric housing codes increasingly have failed to adopt requirements related to health. For example, radon mitigation is an optional appendix to the International Residential Code. The International Code Council consistently failed to adopt safe lead work practices in its maintenance codes for more than a decade. Despite these deficiencies, many housing and building codes, such as the International Property Maintenance Code, have important requirements that can improve public health (National Center for Healthy Housing 2010).

During the 1990s, attention returned to how housing conditions affect public health, as the lead poisoning prevention programs in the United States advanced, and as the EPA launched new initiatives around the indoor environment and radon in particular. In the United Kingdom, work began on a Healthy Housing Rating System originating from work done in the late 1980s (Office of the Deputy Prime Minister 2004). In the United States, HUD, together with the CDC, sent a report to Congress in 1999, launching the nation's healthy homes initiative (HUD 2009). This report focused initially on mold and moisture control, ventilation, dust control, and education. The U.S. Congress provided financial support for this initiative.

In the years immediately following 2000, healthy homes' infrastructure development and research accelerated. The CDC, with support from HUD, launched the National Healthy Homes Training Center and Network. Anchored by the National Center for Healthy Housing, thousands of healthy homes practitioners as of this writing have been trained through a network of 27 universities and institutions. Completion of a course and examination now results in a credential offered through the National Environmental Health Association. In Britain, an extensive training operation resulted in a new protocol now in place for the majority of the nation's housing inspectorate. Globally, the World Health Organization conducted important conferences in 2004–2005, and Warwick University in England organized an international conference in 2008, all of which contributed to the growing recognition that healthy housing remains an urgent matter. Other important developments include a *Call to Action to Promote Healthy Homes* from the U.S. Surgeon General in 2009 and a new Healthy Housing Strategic Plan from HUD. A new federal interagency work group on healthy housing includes the CDC, EPA, HUD, and Departments of Energy and Agriculture, among others.

KEY HEALTHY HOUSING PRINCIPLES

The curriculum development efforts in the United States, England, and elsewhere have led to a refinement of healthy homes principles. Such refinement is likely to continue in coming years. At the time of this writing, the seven key principles can be stated as follows:

To be healthy, a house should be kept:
- dry: free of excessive moisture and leaks;
- ventilated: with both fresh air and proper air distribution and exhaust;
- contaminant-free: free of lead, radon, and certain organic compounds, such as formaldehyde and others;
- pest-free;
- clean;
- maintained; and
- safe: from injury hazards (see Chapter 3).

This listing of key principles is not an exhaustive one. For example, some have proposed that other important features of a healthy home should include adequate lighting, accessibility, comfort, proper density, proper housing amenities for the elderly, and other issues.

The first step in making a home healthy is to determine what hazards are present, which requires an on-site inspection, usually a visual one. Several different protocols and "checklists" have been published to aid in the inspection process. Two leading protocols include the CDC/HUD *Healthy Housing Inspection Manual* (2007) and *The Pediatric Environmental Home Assessment* (National Center for Healthy Housing 2009).

Any checklist or inspection protocol will need to be adapted to specific housing conditions in the locality. Further details on these items can be found in the CDC/HUD *Healthy Housing Inspection Manual* (2007).

MOISTURE

Health Concerns Related to Excessive Moisture in Housing

Excessive moisture in housing has been related to numerous adverse health outcomes in both the general and especially vulnerable segments of the population, such as immunocompromised individuals. Aside from the obvious physical injury hazards associated with structural rot, rust, and other degradation, as well as slips or falls from slippery surfaces, moisture in housing has been associated with asthma, upper respiratory tract symptoms, and other mold-induced illnesses (caused by the increase in biologic agents linked to asthma exacerbation, e.g., dust mites and pest intrusion); communicable diseases associated with poor sanitation; and childhood lead poisoning caused by deteriorated lead paint (Institute of Medicine 2000, 2004). There is also suggestive evidence that mold exposure is associated with airflow obstruction (in otherwise healthy persons), mucous membrane irritation, and pulmonary hemorrhage in infants (Pestka et al. 2008). Around 21% of current asthma cases are believed to be associated with dampness and mold exposure in housing (Dales et al. 2008).

Moisture is connected to household pests. For example, German and American cockroaches are attracted to warm, humid areas near water heaters, laundry areas, bathrooms, appliances, and plumbing fixtures, whereas the Oriental cockroach prefers damp areas such as basements, plumbing, and sewers (Eggleston and Arruda 2001). Dust mites absorb all their water from the air, therefore houses that have a consistent relative humidity more than 50% may have higher levels of dust mites (Arlian et al. 1992).

Molds (fungi) obtain nutrients and moisture for growth from water-affected building materials such as wallboard and insulation materials, as well as carpets, furniture, and bedding (Institute of Medicine 2004). Mold exposure occurs primarily as spores become aerosolized. Exposure to indoor molds is potentially widespread, because they are ubiquitous. The National Survey of Lead and Allergens in Housing found that 56% of homes had levels of some molds above the threshold associated with asthma symptoms (Salo et al. 2008), although no exposure limits for mold have been developed.

People exposed to more allergens are more likely to become sensitized, especially those with asthma or born to atopic mothers (Illi et al. 2006). Reducing moisture and removing moldy items benefit health. One study of 164 homes showed that eradication of visible mold through removal, fungicide application, and ventilation fan installation reduced symptoms and medication use among people with asthma (Burr et al. 2007). Another smaller study (Kercsmar et al. 2006) showed improved clinical outcomes with decreased exposure to mold. Exposure to dust mite allergen is also associated with asthma exacerbations, and asthmatic symptoms improve when dust mite allergens are reduced (Platts-Mills and Mitchell 1982).

Measuring Moisture Levels in Homes

Apart from floods, sources of water and moisture in homes include structural leaks (e.g., roof leaks), condensation, damp foundations and crawl spaces, inadequate ventilation, activities such as bathing and cooking, and plumbing leaks (Dales et al. 2008). Condensation is often linked to inadequate vapor barriers or poor ventilation. Building envelopes that are "tightened" for energy-conservation purposes may sometimes lead to excessive indoor moisture levels unless sufficient fresh, tempered air is brought into the living space.

Moisture measurements can be obtained in numerous ways and are instructive in identifying locations needing attention. Relative humidity, expressed as a percentage value, is a measure of the amount of water vapor in the air (at a specific temperature) compared with the maximum amount of water vapor that air could hold at that temperature. Relative humidity depends on the temperature of the air, because warm air can hold more moisture than cold air. A relative humidity of 100% indicates that the air is holding all the water it can at the current temperature, and any additional moisture at that point will result in condensation. A relative humidity of 50% means the air is holding half the amount of moisture that it could. As the temperature decreases, the amount of moisture in the air does not change, but the relative humidity goes up (because the maximum amount of moisture that cooler air can hold is smaller). Interior moisture levels are typically dependent to some extent on exterior weather, making a uniform definition of acceptable interior moisture levels dependent on different climate zones. In general, maintaining an indoor relative humidity between 30% and 50% can be expected to optimize health (American Society of Heating, Refrigerating, and Air-Conditioning Engineers 2001).

Relative humidity is measured with hygrometers. One of the simplest types of hygrometers is the sling psychrometer, which is simply two thermometers: one is open to the air, and the other is housed in a moistened sock. As the psychrometer is moved through the air, the dry bulb reading can be compared with the wet bulb reading (as the water evaporates from the sock, it cools the surface, much as perspiration in the human body keeps a person cool). A simple formula is then used to calculate the percent relative humidity.

It is also possible to measure the water content (more properly termed "water activity") of building components, but there are no established standards for how much moisture content can be expected for different materials. For example, the ability of drywall to hold water is very different from that of plaster or concrete. Moisture meters are also available that measure water content in air or building materials through measuring changes in electrical resistance/capacitance. Two major kinds of moisture meters include those that measure surface moisture through measuring current between two electrodes and those that have two pins that can be inserted into building materials to measure moisture content or water activity (Figure 2.1).

Two other methods exist for identifying interior moisture problems: thermography and direct observation. Thermography involves the use of sophisticated infrared imaging to "see" areas that have high moisture content. Areas with high moisture are typically cooler than dry areas, and sensing technology is now sufficiently advanced such that areas enclosed or not otherwise visible can be observed through the infrared spectrum. Because infrared radiation is emitted by all objects according to their temperatures, thermography makes it possible to "see" one's environment with or without visible illumination. The amount of radiation emitted by an object increases with temperature, which means that thermography enables the observation of variations in temperature.

Moisture problems can often be assessed easily through direct observation by trained individuals. The CDC/HUD *Healthy Housing Inspection Manual* (2007) calls for identification of moisture-related building deficiencies such as discolored ceiling tiles; presence of visible condensation; missing or damaged downspouts and gutters; presence of holes or cracks in building walls; plumbing systems that have inadequately

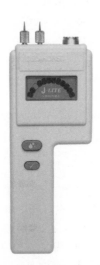

Source: Courtesy of Delmhorst Instrument Co.

Figure 2.1 — Handheld 2-pin moisture meter.

insulated cold water pipes (leading to condensation); and sewage, water drain, and supply leaks. Many housing moisture problems can be readily assessed through observation.

Remediation of Housing Moisture Problems

Ventilation and dehumidification are generally useful in reducing humidity levels. A national survey found that the use of a dehumidifier was an independent predictor of lower levels of some asthma triggers and mold (Salo et al. 2005). Also, installation of whole-house mechanical ventilation can decrease humidity, mite numbers, and mite allergen levels, as well as improve clinical outcomes (Warner et al. 2000). Dehumidification in temperate climates with air conditioners and dehumidifiers is effective (Arlian et al. 2002). Ventilation and moisture control are typically related, and ventilation also can decrease indoor contaminants (assuming the outdoor supply air has lower levels of contaminants than the indoor air, which is not always the case, e.g., location of housing near point sources such as industrial emissions and high traffic roadways). In high-humidity climates, whole-house ventilation has been less effective (Crane et al. 1998; Niven et al. 1999).

Drying and Dehumidification

If the housing has become too wet, drying the affected area is usually the first step following identification and correction of the source. However, some forms of drying can make the problem worse. For example, blowing high-velocity air streams over surfaces contaminated with extensive mold can cause mold spores and fragments to become airborne, where they can be readily inhaled or contaminate other surfaces. Use of dehumidifiers, proper personal protection, and other measures can help to avoid these problems. In some cases, it may be necessary to dispose of contaminated items that cannot be properly cleaned. Mold and moisture remediation guidelines are available from the EPA (2002) and the American Industrial Hygiene Association (2008). If the damage is extensive, a trained professional should be employed to address the problem.

How Ventilation Can Affect Moisture

For some moisture problems, changes to the house ventilation system may be needed. For example, a ventilation system that draws in supply air from a moist basement, instead of from a tempered living area or fresh outdoor air may result in dispersal of moisture and mold throughout the house. A simple solution is to run a duct from the supply air intake to the exterior or to a tempered living area (Figure 2.2).

Houses equipped with air conditioning or dehumidifying systems require attention to ensure that condensate drains do not become blocked. Such blockage can

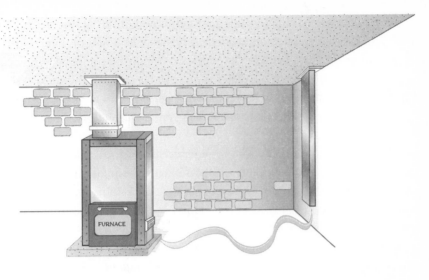

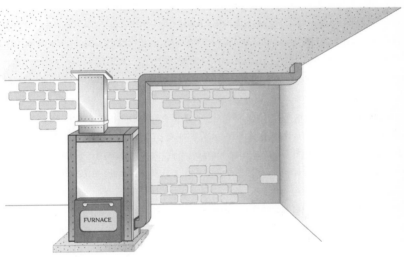

Source: Courtesy of Environmental Health Watch.

Figure 2.2—Ventilation. Top, improper air supply. Bottom, proper air supply.

result in leaks from the drainage pans onto other surfaces that in some cases may not be directly visible. Condensate drains should be checked regularly and cleaned as needed. In addition, condensate pans need to be properly sloped so that the water runs to the drain and does not pool in other areas. Cooling coils also need to be cleaned to prevent blockage and higher fuel consumption caused by lower heat transfer.

Some heating, ventilation, and air-conditioning (HVAC) systems are equipped with humidifiers, especially in northern climates where indoor winter air can become quite dry. In other cases, specific rooms may be equipped with local humidifiers. In both cases, the water supply, water tank, and water wheels or other distribution systems need to be kept clean. If the systems are not used for some time, they can become breeding grounds for biological agents, including mold, bacteria, and viruses.

Another system that can lead to moisture problems if not present or not properly installed and maintained is local exhaust ventilation for high moisture areas, such as bathrooms and kitchens. Many codes do not require such systems if windows are present. Of course, if windows are not opened during peak water use (e.g., bathing), which is often the case when the outdoors is too cold or hot, then moisture will have nowhere to go other than the rest of the living area. Kitchens can also benefit from such local exhaust in removing not only excess moisture but also combustion gases from fuel-fired stoves and ovens, which can release carbon monoxide (CO), oxides of nitrogen, and other dangerous combustion by-products. New and rehabilitated houses are increasingly being equipped with humidistats that automatically operate the exhaust fans when moisture increases to a certain level, which conserves energy as well as eliminates reliance on behavior.

When installing exhaust ventilation for kitchens and baths, the issue of supply air matters. If makeup (fresh) air is not provided, then air flow will be lower or nonexistent, or even worse, may cause reverse air flow in chimneys, hot water heaters, and other devices that can release dangerous gases into the living area.

Exterior Grading and Poolings

A common point of water penetration into a building often occurs at the foundation and ground level. Evidence of standing water, pooling, or erosion means that the soil and ground around the foundation are not properly sloped and graded. Maintaining proper grading around a foundation helps prevent the need for expensive foundation waterproofing and excavation, as well as moisture intrusion into basements. This also promotes the durability of the structure by reducing the prospect of settling, which often leads to cracks. For new construction, installing capillary breaks around interior foundation walls helps avoid water being "wicked" up from the ground and into the building through capillary action.

Vapor Barriers

Vapor barriers are needed for areas prone to high moisture levels and high temperature differentials, such as crawl spaces, attics, and exterior walls. Proper installation is dependent on climate zones and specific building factors. Improper installation could cause the insulation behind the vapor barrier to accumulate moisture from condensation, resulting in a mold problem. Similarly, cold water pipes located in areas where the air is warm (or hot water pipes located in areas where the air is cold) should be insulated to prevent condensation. One way of detecting this problem is to look for runs of discoloration where condensate from pipes has dripped onto a lower surface, such as ceiling tiles. The same principle applies to duct work that carries warm or cold air through air zones with a high temperature gradient. Duct work should be sealed and well insulated to prevent such condensation, and the insulation should be applied to the exterior of the duct work, not the interior. Interior insulation can become breeding grounds for mold and other biological agents.

Flashing

A common building deficiency associated with leakage of water through the building envelope is the absence (or deterioration) of flashing. Flashing refers to thin, continuous pieces of sheet metal or other impervious material installed to prevent the passage of water into a structure through an angle or joint. It operates on the principle that, for water to penetrate a joint, it must work itself upward against the force of gravity or wind-driven rain. Flashing may be exposed or concealed. Exposed flashing is usually sheet metal, such as aluminum, copper, painted galvanized steel, stainless steel, zinc alloy, terne metal, lead, or lead-coated copper. Metal flashing should be provided with expansion joints on long runs to prevent deformation of the metal sheets. The selected metal should not stain or be stained by adjacent materials or react chemically with them.

Flashing concealed within a construction assembly may be sheet metal or a waterproofing membrane such as bituminous fabric or plastic sheet material, depending on the climate and structural requirements. Aluminum can react chemically with cement mortar, and some flashing materials can deteriorate with exposure to sunlight.

Flashing has many forms—roof penetrations such as chimneys, walls, windows, and other structural discontinuities. When new building assemblies, such as windows, are installed, they should be accompanied by flashing to prevent unwanted moisture incursion. Flashing at the base of structures should have "weep holes" to allow water that has been repelled by the flashing a way to escape the plane of the building surface. The principle of flashing should be extended to all penetrations in structures, that is, they should be sealed to prevent moisture (and pest) incursion into the living area.

Windows and Condensation

Window condensation also deserves special consideration. It depends on the indoor and outdoor temperature and humidity levels. Condensation most often occurs on windows because they traditionally are not adequately insulated. Modern double- and triple-pane windows, some filled with inert gases between the panes, effectively eliminate condensation problems when properly configured for the specific building application, orientation, and climate. Replacing traditional windows with more modern configurations has the benefit of removing a major source of lead poisoning as well. Old single-pane windows are known to have the highest levels of lead-contaminated dust and paint of any other building component (Jacobs et al. 2002).

Drains

As important as entry of excess moisture into a building is, attention must also be given to how it leaves. Drains are often overlooked as important sources of moisture, as leaks from them may be slow. Drain traps can also become degraded over time. If drain traps are not kept full of water, harmful soil gases can enter the living area. Basement-floor drain traps should be kept full by periodically dumping water into them.

Education

Occupant behavior can have a strong influence on interior moisture levels. Prompt reporting of leaks and condensation, use of exhaust ventilation to remove moisture, and maintenance of equipment such as humidifiers, dehumidifiers, and drains should be a part of all resident training programs and homeowner education. Water issues sometimes are regarded as a cosmetic or small matter (with the exception of a large leak or disaster-related water incursion) instead of a very real health problem if not properly and swiftly addressed.

VENTILATION

Most homes in the United States do not have a planned supply of fresh air delivered to the building space, instead relying on windows, doors, and intermittent or inadequate building leakage. Thus, indoor airborne contaminants can increase. Indoor chemicals in the home environment can include lead, pesticides, environmental tobacco smoke (ETS), CO, volatile organic compounds (VOCs), radon, and others. Exposure to high levels of CO has been associated with fatalities. Indoor chemical agents are known to be related to health problems in the brain and nervous system, developmental disorders, asthma and other respiratory illnesses, and cancer and other illnesses (reviewed in Jacobs and Baeder 2009). Structural deficiencies, pest infestations, gas stoves, and the introduction of source materials that off-gas or otherwise release toxic agents are all housing factors that can increase the presence of chemical agents in or around a dwelling. Methods of measuring airborne contaminants have been well described (CDC/HUD 2007).

Secondhand Smoke

The U.S. EPA (1992) states that secondhand smoke causes approximately 3,000 lung cancer deaths in nonsmokers each year, not to mention the thousands more who are affected as smokers. Exposure to tobacco smoke also has been associated with premature birth, low birth weight, low Apgar scores, poor early growth of infants, and dysfunctional behavior (Bauman, Flewelling, and LaPrelle 1991; Eskenazi and Trupin 1995; Fergusson, Horwood, and Lynskey 1993; Williams et al. 1998). Secondhand smoke is a complex mixture of 4,000 chemicals, at least 40 of which cause cancer; others can also irritate the respiratory system and affect other organs (U.S. EPA 1992). The Surgeon General's report (Office of the Surgeon General 2006), *The Health Consequences of Involuntary Exposure to Tobacco Smoke*, found that children exposed to secondhand smoke are at greater risk for sudden infant death syndrome, acute respiratory disease, ear problems, and more severe asthma episodes. The report concluded that there is no risk-free level of exposure to secondhand smoke.

Carbon Monoxide

Sixty-four percent of nonfatal CO exposures occur in the home (CDC 2005). The main sources of CO in the home include malfunctioning or inadequately vented gas appliances, oil or wood-burning appliances, tobacco smoke, and unvented appliances that are designed for outdoor use, such as gasoline-powered electricity generators. Hundreds of deaths and thousands of nonfatal poisonings occur annually in the United States from CO (CDC 2005). Both acute (short-term exposures to high concentrations of CO) and chronic (lower-level, repeated) exposures have serious health effects. Survivors of CO poisoning may have long-term neurologic effects, such as personality changes, memory deficits, impaired judgment, poor concentration, and other adverse health effects (U.S. EPA 2001).

Pesticides

Pesticides are any substance used to suppress pests. Exposure to pesticides can occur through diet, dermal absorption, and inhalation of airborne pesticides as an aerosol or adsorbed on dust particles (Institute of Medicine 2000). In 2000, 75% of U.S. households used at least one pesticide indoors during the past year, and 80% of most people's exposure to pesticides occurred indoors (U.S. EPA 2004). Pesticides are a particular concern for low-income neighborhoods, whether urban or rural, where pest infestations (e.g., cockroaches, mice, and rats) are common (Berkowitz et al. 2003; Whyatt et al. 2002). Pesticides can remain in a home for years after use has stopped and have been found in indoor air, in carpet dust, and on settled dust surfaces. Inert ingredients, not typically included in risk assessments, are also potentially hazardous and may contribute to the effects from the active ingredients (Watson et al. 2003). For example, some "inert ingredients" are actually volatile organic solvents. Pesticides often target the nervous system, and there may be a cumulative risk from exposure to multiple pesticides (Eskenazi et al. 2008).

Volatile Organic Compounds

VOCs are gases at normal room temperature and pressure. Common household items that can release VOCs include paint, varnish, and wax; cleaning, disinfecting, cosmetic, and degreasing products; products containing particle board and plywood; so-called air fresheners; and hobby products. VOCs that commonly pollute indoor air include toluene, styrene, xylene, benzene, trichloroethylene, formaldehyde, and other aldehydes. Semi-volatile compounds, such as phthalates, may also be harmful. The health effects of VOCs are varied. Elevated indoor concentrations of VOC mixtures may play a role in the constellation of symptoms known as "sick building syndrome" (e.g., headaches, fatigue, and eye and upper respiratory irritation). Formaldehyde is a component of some building materials, such as particle board and plywood adhesives, and may be found at high levels in new buildings or new furniture where formaldehyde and other aldehydes are used in the binding agent. Some VOCs, such as formaldehyde, can also produce sensitization, such that subsequent low-level exposures trigger significant health problems.

Radon

Exposure to radon—an odorless, tasteless, radioactive, and naturally occurring gas—is the leading cause of lung cancer among nonsmokers and the second leading cause of lung cancer overall. Exposure to radon causes 21,000 deaths annually in the United States (U.S. EPA 2003). Combined data from several previous residential studies show definitive evidence of an association between residential radon exposure and lung cancer (Darby 2005; Krewski et al. 2006; Samet 2006). Radon can enter houses through fractures and porous substrates in the foundations of buildings and can be highly concentrated in certain areas. Radon may also enter a house through water systems in communities where groundwater is the main water supply. This is most common in small public systems and private wells that are typically closed systems and do not allow radon to escape. Housing with high radon concentrations is more prevalent in certain regions of the country, but any house, regardless of region, can contain dangerous or unhealthy levels of radon. The EPA has a map of high-risk radon areas (U.S. EPA 1993).

Types of Housing Ventilation

Good ventilation can help keep exposures to contaminants, odors, moisture, and other substance quite low. However, controlling the source of the contaminant is always the primary approach, because ventilation cannot always be expected to keep exposures low. If a contaminant exists in a home, its source should be investigated and determined before a ventilation system is installed or otherwise improved.

Ventilation systems generally fall into two categories: local exhaust ventilation and general dilution ventilation. Local exhaust ventilation moves a relatively small amount of air to remove a contaminant at the point it is generated, before it can enter the indoor air at large. Examples in the home include kitchen and bathroom exhaust, chimneys, clothes driers, and vented combustion appliances (furnaces, hot water heaters). General dilution ventilation moves larger volumes of air and, as the name implies, dilutes contaminants with uncontaminated air. Many homes do not have a planned fresh air supply. Instead, whatever fresh air is delivered tends to come through building leakage, opening windows and doors, or in some cases "whole-house ventilation," such as attic exhaust systems. As building envelopes are tightened for energy conservation purposes and building leakage declines, it is vital that an adequate supply of fresh air be planned and installed. One study in California showed that windows are used far less often than previously thought (Offerman 2009).

Air-flow patterns can be complex and may flow in unexpected directions. Generally, air moves from high to low pressure and warm air rises while cold air settles. All buildings have a "stack effect," which is caused by air buoyancy. For example, hot air flows up through a chimney. In tall buildings, this can sometimes cause apartments on the lower floors to be cold, while those on the upper floors are hot. Regulating pressure differentials so that air moves as intended is essential to good building design. Failure to regulate these pressure differentials can have disastrous consequences. For example, if a new exhaust system is added without balancing air pressure, air that would normally rise through a chimney or fireplace can actually reverse direction and enter the living area, bringing CO and other contaminants with it.

Methods of Detecting Ventilation and Air Flow

Many tools are available to measure ventilation and air flow. This section focuses on four simple methods that can identify problems. Smoke tubes or smoke bottles are made of nontoxic chemicals. When the smoke is released, it can be watched to see how the air is moving. This method is often used to determine whether kitchen and bath exhaust systems are working, chimneys have sufficient draw, or air flow has been reversed. The method can also help identify the influence of opening or closing windows and doors on ventilation and air flow.

A more quantitative approach involves the use of instruments, such as velometers, anemometers, or pitot tubes. Velometers measure the speed of air flow, usually in feet per second. They often do not require a power source and operate by a swinging vane, which is a plate that is depressed as the air presses against it. Velometers are typically used to measure the speed of air (face velocity) at openings into which air moves, such as an exhaust or supply air opening. A similar device is an anemometer, which also measures air speed, typically by the cooling effect of air moving across a heated wire. The faster the air, the greater the cooling effect. This type of device can be used to measure air flow inside duct work, which often involves drilling a hole into the duct. A third type of device is a pitot tube, which is a tube set parallel to the air flow direction. Small holes are located in the end and side of the tube, which has hoses attached to a manometer to measure pressure differentials. A pitot tube enables one to quantify air speed, total and static pressure, and other factors.

A third device is a flow capture hood. This instrument measures air flow in cubic feet per minute (cfm) and typically has an opening that is placed over an exhaust or supply air vent. There are a series of pitot tubes or electronic sensors that measure air speed; because the dimensions of the hood are known, it is possible to obtain volumetric air flows as well (Figure 2.3).

Many ventilation system problems can be identified visually. For example, looking for discoloration under doors suggests that air pressure differentials

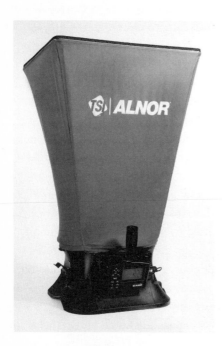

Source: Courtesy of TSI Incorporated.

Figure 2.3 — Flow capture hood.

between the two rooms may be too high. Pooling or ponding of water near air intakes may cause unnecessary moisture to infiltrate the building. If an attached garage is present and the doors are not sealed, it is possible for CO and VOCs to enter the living space. If an exhaust vent is located too close to a supply vent, the air can be "short-circuited": instead of mixing with the supply air and diluting the contaminants, air enters the room and is immediately exhausted. Visual inspection can also identify incorrect ducting problems (too many twists and turns), disconnected ducts, and misaligned chimney and hot water flues.

Ventilation systems should be "balanced." This means that duct runs and fans should be properly sized to operate as designed. This is usually done during initial construction and may be part of a final commissioning step required by some green building programs.

Specific Ventilation Controls
SOURCE CONTROL

Common deficiencies leading to health problems often can be corrected by installing proper ventilation. As described earlier, source control should always be the first step. For example, building materials, carpeting, and furnishings that do not off-gas formaldehyde or other VOCs should be used instead of those that do. Although some countries require testing of building materials before they can be sold, the United States currently does not do so routinely.

RADON

Radon mitigation systems are varied, requiring a trained and licensed contractor for proper installation. Active radon sub-slab depressurization is perhaps the most involved (and most effective) system. Briefly, it consists of a pipe that is punched through the concrete slab in the basement or foundation. The other end of the pipe is routed through the building and out through the roof. The pipe has a fan and equipment to monitor the fan's operation. As the fan pulls air through the pipe, it depressurizes the soil underneath the foundation so that instead of allowing radon to enter the building, it is exhausted out through the roof. Merely sealing the basement may not be adequate because of the stack effect and because most buildings are under negative pressure with respect to the exterior. A "passive" form of radon sub-slab depressurization is the pipe without the fan. This system may not be effective in consistently reducing indoor radon levels to less than 4 pCi/L, the current EPA exposure limit. These systems are described in greater detail in another publication (U.S. EPA 2010).

For new construction, it is possible to seal foundations so that radon is unlikely to reach high levels indoors. Radon-resistant new construction measures should always be implemented in EPA Zones 1 and 2 on the radon map (U.S. EPA 1993). The techniques involve the use of gas-impermeable membranes at the foundation and sealing of all penetrations.

There is substantial evidence that active radon mitigation is effective (Brodhead 1995; Groves-Kirkby et al. 2006; Huber, Ennemoser, and Schneider 2001; Tuccillo and Rauch 1994). Each of these studies enrolled a relatively large number of housing units, ranging from 73 to 238 units. In particular, the studies by Groves-Kirkby et al. and Burkhart and Kladder had well-characterized control groups and were able to demonstrate significant reductions in radon exposures using active soil depressurization systems. Groves-Kirkby et al. showed that active soil depressurization systems were far more effective than installation of membranes during construction. An EPA review concluded that 97% of houses with high baseline radon levels (76% had baseline radon levels ≥ 10 pCi/L) could be remediated with active soil depressurization systems to less than 4 pCi/L (Burkhart and Kladder 1991). The Brodhead study (1995), which was a national survey, showed that 95% of remediated homes had radon levels less than 4 pCi/L and that 69% actually had levels less than 2 pCi/L (n = 238 houses).

In some circumstances, radon in drinking water may be a concern. Further information on methods of remediating radon in drinking water is available at http://www.epa.gov/radon.

LOCAL EXHAUST VENTILATION

All kitchens and bathrooms should be equipped with exhaust systems to remove moisture and odors.Quiet ENERGY STAR fans should be installed, because a noisy, high-energy fan is less likely to be used consistently. The fans should be attached to ducts to exhaust outside the building envelope, not inside a wall cavity where mold could grow. The American Society of Heating Refrigeration and Air-Conditioning Engineers (ASHRAE) recommends that kitchen fans exhaust 100 cfm and bathroom fans exhaust 50 cfm. Actual fan performance will depend on the duct configuration and other factors that contribute to pressure drops (resistance) in the system. For example, a fan rated at 50 cfm located in a basement bathroom that has to push air through several stories before being exhausted may not move as much air as needed. In other words, the fan needs to be sized to fit the building configuration.

When installing exhaust ventilation for kitchens and baths, the issue of supply (makeup) air matters. If makeup air is not provided, air flow will be lower or nonexistent, or may cause reverse air flow in chimneys, hot water heaters, and other devices that can release dangerous gases into the living area.

All clothes driers should also be exhausted to the exterior; energy-conservation devices that permit warm, moist air from clothes drier exhaust to be recirculated back into the house should not be used. All combustion burning appliances, such as fuel-fired space heaters, should also be exhausted to the exterior.

People die of CO poisoning operating electric generators indoors that are meant for outside use. Fuel-burning appliances meant for exterior use should not be brought into the interior.

DILUTION VENTILATION

House ventilation systems first should ensure that the supply air is contaminant-free and does not pass over standing water, automobile garages, or high traffic areas. In some areas, chemical filtration may be needed in addition to the usual particulate filters that are installed. Air filters in ventilation systems need to be changed frequently so that the pressure drop across the filter does not become too great, thus reducing air flow. Furnace filters that are more efficient at removing small particles are now available.

When dilution ventilation systems are designed or retrofitted, they should comply with ASHRAE 62 (62.1 is the standard for multifamily buildings, and 62.2 is the standard for low-rise and single-family dwellings). The ASHRAE standard has two features—it determines the amount of fresh air that is needed according to both the size of the building (to control off-gassing) and the number of people who occupy the space. Because most buildings currently bring in lower air flows than those specified by ASHRAE, increasing the air flow could result in an energy penalty, unless the energy in the exhaust air is captured and used to temper the supply air. High-efficiency air exchangers are now available, avoiding the need to trade off good air quality with low energy costs and carbon emissions.

PORTABLE AIR CLEANERS

The ability of air cleaners to remove particulate matter of certain size ranges from air is well established. Specifically, air cleaners are known to be able to achieve a 30%–70% reduction in the half-life of airborne particulate matter between 0.3 and 1 µm (Batterman, Godwin, and Jia 2005). However, Batterman, Godwin, and Jia also showed that air cleaners did not reduce larger airborne particles (1–5 µm). Air cleaners are less effective as the particle size increases, and they have not been demonstrated to reduce VOCs or other gases, such as CO, oxides of nitrogen, and others (Shaughnessy and Sextro 2006). This led the National Academy of Sciences to conclude that there is only limited evidence that air cleaners are effective in reducing asthma (Institute of Medicine 2000). Portable high-efficiency particulate air (HEPA) cleaning devices are capable of greatly reducing very small particles in the indoor environment during forest fires and wood burning (Barn et al. 2008). However, these systems cannot adequately control exposures to ETS; source control through smoking cessation is the only effective solution.

Some so-called air cleaners emit high levels of ozone under the theory that this reactive gas will clean the air. However, exposures to ozone should always be avoided, and these devices should not be used in the home environment. Ozone exposure is associated with asthma morbidity (Trasande and Thurston 2005), and the benefits such devices have on removal of indoor airborne particulate matter are not known (Diette et al. 2008).

PEST INFESTATIONS

Pests in housing are associated with many adverse health effects and exposures. Pests have been recognized to be carriers of disease for centuries. The traditional method of addressing pests has been trapping or poisoning. In keeping with the key principles of healthy housing, a broader approach is presented here that has demonstrated widespread success.

The evidence linking mites, cockroaches, and rodents with asthma is substantial. The Institute of Medicine found sufficient evidence to establish a causal association between asthma incidence and dust mite exposure and between asthma exacerbations and the presence of dust mites, cockroaches, and pet dander (Institute of Medicine 2000). The body parts and excreta that these organisms shed release proteins and other chemicals known collectively as allergens, which are strongly associated with asthma and other respiratory and allergic health problems. Rodents that shed skin and other proteins may also be an important indoor allergen affecting inner-city and suburban children with asthma (Dales et al. 2008; Matsui et al. 2003; Phipatanakul et al. 2000). Cockroach allergens are an important cause of asthma exacerbations, particularly in deteriorated homes where cockroach infestation is most common (Chew et al. 2008; Rauh, Ches, and Garfinkel 2002). The National Cooperative Inner City Asthma Study (a multisite intervention study in the United States) found that among a group of inner-city children, cockroach allergens had a greater effect on asthma morbidity than dust mites or pet allergens (Gruchalla et al. 2005). Cockroaches may also be an important factor in asthma exacerbation in rural and suburban homes (Matsui et al. 2003). A detectable level of cockroach allergen has been found in 63% of dwellings in the United States (Cohn 2006), and 10.2% of all dwellings have cockroach allergen levels above the asthma morbidity threshold (Salo et al. 2008). National data show that high concentrations of cockroach allergen are associated with high-rise buildings, urban settings, pre-1940 construction, and household incomes less than $20,000 (Cohn 2006). A recent survey found that more than 80% of homes in the United States had detectable levels of house dust mite allergen in the bedroom, 46% had levels associated with sensitization, and 24% had levels associated with asthma (Arbes Jr., Cohn, et al. 2003).

In addition to these exposures, residents can also be exposed to fungicides, insecticides, rodenticides, cleaning agents, poisons, and other chemicals that are used to eradicate pest infestations. Failure to address pests can lead to a host of communicable diseases, bites, and infections, and, if not addressed, to fatalities. The list of potential pests is long, but the most common in the housing environment are rodents (including rats and mice), cockroaches, dust mites, bedbugs, birds, bats, scabies (often associated with dust mites), squirrels, chipmunks and other mammals, mosquitoes, and other insects.

As with the other healthy housing issues, pests in housing and the methods of detecting and controlling them are often intertwined with other housing deficiencies, especially inadequate moisture control and ventilation. Holes and penetrations in the building envelope can permit pests to enter the dwelling. Furthermore, poor moisture control can provide the necessary water for pests' survival, leaving only nutrients as the remaining need. Access to nutrients can often be prevented by proper storage of food, trash, and garbage, along with cleaning food-preparation surfaces, utensils, and other equipment.

Detection Methods

Methods of detecting pests are varied and described in detail in the CDC manual on integrated pest management (IPM) (CDC 2006) (http://www.cdc.gov/nceh/ehs/docs/IPM_Manual.pdf). Visual evidence of pest presence is the simplest of these. A trained observer can identify fecal matter released by insects and rodents along common pathways around the perimeters of rooms. Fecal matter from insects is typically spherical, whereas fecal matter from rats or mice is often elongated because of the presence of a sphincter. Other body parts may also be visible, and of course, the most obvious visual evidence is alive or dead pests themselves. Rub marks and burrows are also signs of pest activity. Exterior evidence may include ant mounds, burrows, nests, and so forth. A trained observer looks in food storage areas, trash, and garbage disposal systems, such as trash chutes and trash cans. Penetrations in walls, under kitchen sinks, in basements, and in other areas should all be observed for evidence of pest infestations. Some practitioners have found that the use of a heat gun can drive hidden pests into the open. A visual survey can identify potential harborage sites. Harborage simply means those areas where pests may be able to take shelter, for example, unused boxes in basements, clutter, brush and bushes near structures, and standing water containers. The time of a pest inspection is also important, because some types of pests are most likely to be observed in the evening (cockroaches) (Figure 2.4).

Integrated Pest Management

IPM is a decision-making process that manages the environment to control pests and disease vectors (CDC 2006). As such, it is a departure from the traditional practice of trapping, spraying, and poisoning. If IPM is to be successful, it must consider the behavior and ecology of the specific pest, exactly where it is active, and how environmental changes may influence the pest. IPM includes a strong educational component, because the environment includes the behavior of residents. In some quarters, housing providers may believe that this education component cannot be sufficiently effective to ensure that pest infestations do not occur. Some believe that if only one resident in an apartment building (or a house in a neighborhood) fails to properly store food, trash, and garbage, the whole approach of IPM cannot work. Although education is indeed a critical component, the evidence to date is that IPM is effective in controlling pests, reducing exposure to pesticides, and reducing long-term costs.

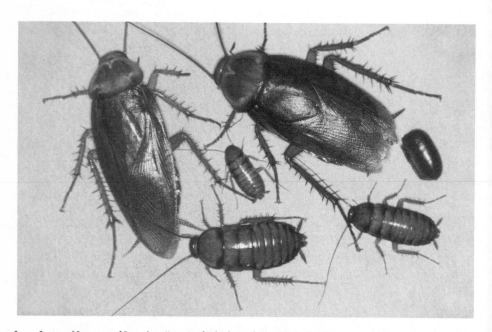

Source: Courtesy of Department of Entomology, University of Nebraska-Lincoln; Jim Kalisch, photographer.

Figure 2.4 — Life stages of the American cockroach (*Periplaneta americana*).

Randomized, controlled studies have demonstrated the effectiveness of IPM in reducing exposure to cockroaches (Arbes, Sever, et al. 2003; Eggleston et al. 2005; Miller and Meek 2004; Wang and Bennett 2006). Arbes, Sever, et al. found that roach allergen levels were significantly reduced in beds and kitchens and that the levels in the beds decreased below the thresholds for both sensitization and exacerbation. Wang and Bennett showed a significantly greater decrease in roach counts with IPM compared with gel bait alone. Miller and Meek found that although IPM was initially more costly, it was much more effective in reducing cockroaches compared with traditional pesticide treatment and is likely to provide significant cost-savings in future years.

A major study showed that both cockroach infestations and levels of pyrethroid insecticides in indoor air samples decreased significantly ($P = .016$) compared with a control group (Williams 2006). In addition, pesticides were not detected in the maternal blood samples. In short, the efficacy of IPM as a means of controlling exposure to pests and their allergens is now well established.

Pets

Although pets are an integral part of many families and cannot be confused with pests, cats, dogs, mice, reptiles, and pet rodents may pose health threats as well as confer health benefits. Individuals concerned about bites, pet dander, or asthmatic exacerbation should read the CDC document on pets (http://www.cdc.gov/healthypets).

CLEANING AND MAINTENANCE

Two other key healthy housing principles include proper cleaning and maintenance. Without these two ongoing activities, housing systems that were designed to prevent injury and ill health will eventually fail, creating new hazards that may not be recognized until harm has occurred. In rental housing, cleaning is typically the responsibility of the occupant (except for common areas in multifamily housing), and maintenance is typically the responsibility of the owner.

The previous sections of this chapter have described a number of conditions that require correction if a home is to be healthy. For example, if one were to repair existing leaks in the roof without implementing a system to identify potential leaks before they develop, mold damage may occur before it is recognized. Similarly, if enclosures that prevent exposure to lead-based paint fall into disrepair, lead paint that previously did not present a hazard could become one if the enclosure fails. Condensate drainage systems that are not kept clean can fail, also leading to mold and moisture problems. Radon mitigation systems can fail if not monitored. Many housing providers have separate budgets and financial resources for maintenance and capital improvements. It is beyond the scope of this book to determine the dividing line between these two, but they are related. Some building systems will become so aged and deteriorated that proper maintenance is no longer feasible or financially viable. In such a case, continuing maintenance without capital improvements will cause an inflated maintenance budget and, more important, cause health problems for the occupants. For owner-occupied, single-family housing, a simple checklist is provided in Table 2.1. For multifamily, large apartment complexes, other schedules with

TABLE 2.1 — NATIONAL CENTER FOR HEALTHY HOUSING MAINTENANCE AND CLEANING CHECKLIST

Yard and Exterior	SPRING	FALL	ANNUAL	AS NEEDED	NEED A PRO?
Water drains away from house	O				
No trip, fall, choking, sharp edge hazards	O	O			
Fence around pool intact	O	O			
Check for signs of rodents, bats, roaches, termites	O	O			
Drain outdoor faucets and hoses		O			
Clean window wells and check drainage	O	O			
Clean gutters and downspouts	O	O			

Basement and Crawlspace	SPRING	FALL	ANNUAL	AS NEEDED	NEED A PRO?
No wet surfaces, puddles	O	O			
Sump pump and check valve working	O	O			
Floor drain working	O				
Vacuum basement surfaces	O				
Check for signs of rodents, bats, roaches, termites			O		

Garage	SPRING	FALL	ANNUAL	AS NEEDED	NEED A PRO?
Ensure storage of fuel cans	O	O			
Proper operation of garage door safety shut-off	O	O			
Check for signs of water damage	O				
Check for signs of rodents, bats, roaches, termites	O	O			

Exterior Roof, Walls, Windows	SPRING	FALL	ANNUAL	AS NEEDED	NEED A PRO?
Shingles in good condition	O				
Check chimney, valley, plumbing vent, skylight flashing	O				
Make sure gutters discharge water away from building	O				
Check attic vents			O		
Check attic for signs of roof leaks	O				
Check for icicles and ice dams				winter	
Look for peeling paint	O				
Look for signs of leaks where deck attaches to house	O				
Check below window and door that flashing is intact	O				
Repair broken, cracked glass			O		
Look for signs of leaks at windows and door sills	O				
Clean dryer vent	O	O			
Check that exhaust ducts are clear	O	O			

Attic	SPRING	FALL	ANNUAL	AS NEEDED	NEED A PRO?
Check for signs of rodents, bats, roaches, termites		O			
Check for water damage		O			
Ensure insulation is in place		O			
Check that fans exhaust to outdoors (check ductwork connections)				O	

TABLE 2.1 — (CONTINUED)

Interior Walls, Ceilings, Windows, Doors	SPRING	FALL	ANNUAL	AS NEEDED	NEED A PROF.
Check for signs of water damage			o		
Check operation of windows and doors	o				
Lubricate and repair windows and doors				o	

Plumbing Fixtures and Appliances	SPRING	FALL	ANNUAL	AS NEEDED	NEED A PROF.
Check washer hoses-connections			o		
Check dishwasher hoses for leaks			o		
Check toilet supply/shut-off valve			o		
Clean and check refrigerator drip pan-icemaker connections			o		
Check shower-tub surrounds for signs of damage			o		
Check traps and drains under sinks, tubs, showers for leaks			o		
Check hot water heater for leaks		o			
Check boiler for leaks		o			
Check water main/meter or well pump for leaks or sweating		o			
Clean septic tank				2 yrs	
Check drain and supply line for leaks	o	o			
Check bath and kitchen fans operation	o	o			

Appliances	SPRING	FALL	ANNUAL	AS NEEDED	NEED A PROF.
Clean kitchen range hood screens				o	
Clean dryer vents and screens	o				
Clean exhaust fan outlets and screens	o				
Clean outdoor intakes and screens		o			
Clean air conditioning coils, drain pans	o				o
Clean dehumidifier coils, check operation	o				
Clean and tune furnaces, boilers, hot water heaters		o			o
Clean and tune ovens and ranges		o			o

Electrical Equipment	SPRING	FALL	ANNUAL	AS NEEDED	NEED A PROF.
Check for damaged cords	o	o			
Test ground fault interrrupters	o				
Test outlets for proper hot, neutral, and ground				once	
Check smoke and CO alarms	o	o			

HVAC Equipment - Replace filters	SPRING	FALL	ANNUAL	AS NEEDED	NEED A PROF.
Warm air furnace (merv 8)		o			
Air conditioner (central air merv 8)	o				
Dehumidifier	o				
Outdoor air to return to heat recovery ventilation		o			

more frequent checks may be needed, depending on the complexity of the building systems and their operation.

Tobacco Smoke

For both single- and multifamily housing, a major factor that influences costs and health is the issue of tobacco smoke. A number of studies from nonresidential settings have shown that smoking bans have been effective in improving health and reducing exposure to ETS (Allwright et al. 2005; Farrelly et al. 2005; Fong et al. 2006; Haw and Gruer 2007). Many green building programs are now including bans on smoking, such as Enterprise Green Community Criteria and Leadership in Energy and Environmental Design.

This checklist is not necessarily exhaustive, but contains the key items that should be examined on a regular basis.

Smooth and Cleanable Surfaces

Difficult-to-clean surfaces, although not hazards themselves, will lay the foundation for a host of other problems. For example, if food preparation surfaces are not smooth, they cannot be adequately cleaned to prevent food-borne communicable diseases. Food particles can become available to pests. Such surfaces may also make the reaccumulation of lead-contaminated dust more likely. As surfaces wear over time, they may become more pitted and difficult to clean. Carpets should not be used in wet areas, such as kitchens, baths, and laundry rooms, because they are more difficult to dry and keep clean. Carpets in other rooms can also act as dust reservoirs if they are not routinely cleaned. The issue of carpets and carpet removal has been the subject of numerous studies, which are reviewed at http://www.nchh. org/Portals/0/Contents/CarpetsHealthyHomes.pdf.

Heating, Ventilation, and Air-Conditioning Systems

All HVAC systems require periodic cleaning and maintenance. Inadequate cleaning may lead to blocked coils, causing mold and higher fuel bills because of energy inefficiency. Condensate drains should be kept clear. Furnace filters should be changed when loaded to permit proper air movement throughout the dwelling and adequate removal of particles. Normally, it is not necessary to clean duct work, because particulate matter that settles inside the ducts is unlikely to become airborne again unless it is disturbed. For unusual circumstances, such as floods, smoke damage, or other contamination, duct cleaning may be necessary for thorough house decontamination. Asbestos may be present in pipe and boiler insulation and other building insulation systems. Unless the insulation becomes friable or is disturbed during maintenance or rehabilitation, it may not present an exposure problem and can be encapsulated.

Cleaning Agents

Some cleaning agents present their own health and safety hazards. Bleach and ammonia compounds are two common cleaning products that can cause severe eye and skin injuries if not handled properly. If bleach and ammonia are mixed, they can also release dangerous gases (e.g., phosgene and other hazardous agents) that can cause severe respiratory injury. Cleaning products should only be used according to the label instructions. If the instructions call for dilution, the undiluted product may cause high exposures, as well as damage to building structures. New "nontoxic" cleaning products are appearing on the market, some carrying "green" or "natural" labeling. Although intuitively appealing, such products may not be any safer than others. Although there are voluntary labeling programs, there are no national standards in place that enable consumers to make truly informed choices. Therefore, a close reading of the product label is essential to the proper use of all cleaning products. If eye contact with cleaning agents does occur, then a full 15-minute immediate rinsing of the eyes is important. Avoidable eye injuries have occurred because injured persons attempted to seek medical attention instead of performing the rinsing, resulting in permanent damage to the eyes en route to the hospital.

Avoidable Uses and Storage of Volatile Organic Compounds

Some products are marked as air fresheners or cleaners that actually add more VOCs to indoor air. At times, such products are used to "cover up" problems that should be solved at the source. For example, use of air fresheners will do nothing to remove a mold problem, and in fact may make it worse, because a false sense of security may be achieved temporarily. Generally, exposures to VOCs, including fragrances and air fresheners, should be minimized to the extent possible.

Similarly, certain storage practices may lead to increased exposures to VOCs. Fuels, gasoline, paint thinners, and paints should be stored in a well-ventilated, exterior location, not inside the home or attached garage. If this is not feasible, then the products should be stored in a location where the doors to the living area have been sealed. In all cases, such substances should be stored in airtight containers. Products that will not be used, such as old paints or banned pesticides, should be disposed of properly.

Prevention of Track-In Dust

Many contaminants are tracked into the house. Lead from soil, pesticides, bacteria, mold, and many other substances can be carried into the home on shoes. Such track-in can be reduced by the use of both exterior and interior floor mats, which need to be cleaned and maintained to be effective. Some households now store shoes at the entryway, as is a common practice in many Asian cultures as a way to maintain interior cleanliness and reduce track-in.

High-Efficiency Particulate Air Vacuums and Central Vacuums

All carpets should be vacuumed periodically. Normal household vacuum cleaners can sometimes emit large quantities of fine particles through the exhaust, which can lead to increased levels of airborne particulate matter. A solution involves the use of HEPA vacuum cleaners is one option, equipped with a special filter to remove nearly all of the small particles from the vacuum exhaust that would otherwise reenter the room air. These vacuums were quite expensive a few years ago but are now

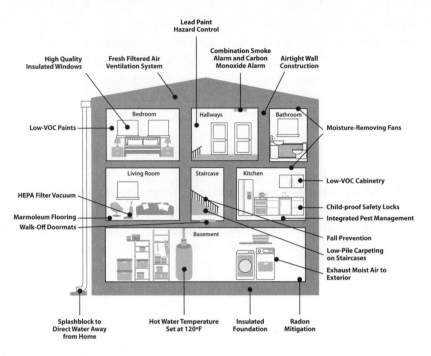

Source: Courtesy of the National Center for Healthy Housing.

Figure 2.5 — Summary of key healthy housing interventions.

more widely available and more affordable. All vacuums used on carpeted floors should be equipped with a beater bar to dislodge bound particulate matter.

A second option is the installation of a central vacuum system in the house, which is filtered and delivers the exhaust air to the outside of the house. Such systems are increasingly finding their way into new construction, although retrofits into existing housing may still be expensive.

Site Maintenance

Maintenance and cleaning operations should apply not only to the interior of the house but also to the exterior and the site. For example, trash storage and pickup locations should be kept clean to avoid attracting pests. Vegetation should be trimmed and maintained to avoid moisture and mildew problems and water ponding on the grounds.

Limitations of Cleaning and Maintenance

Cleaning and maintenance alone will not be sufficient to create healthy housing. Even repeated professional cleaning alone will not prevent childhood lead poisoning from exposure to lead paint hazards (Tohn et al. 2003; Jacobs, Mielke, and Pavur 2003). Removal of pesticide residues will not improve health by itself. The causes of these health hazards must be addressed to assure their prevention.

CONCLUSION

Identifying and correcting housing-related health and safety hazards will not only prevent illnesses and injuries but also support good health. Most of these illnesses and injuries are entirely preventable, and the evidence showing that the interventions are effective is substantial. Investments in healthy homes (Figure 2.5) hold great promise for driving down health care costs and improving the quality of life for all.

REFERENCES

Agency for Toxic Substances and Disease Registry. *Toxicological Profile for Lead*. Washington, DC: U.S. Department of Health and Human Services, 2007. Available at: http://www.atsdr. cdc.gov/toxprofiles/tp13.html.

Allwright, S., G. Paul, B. Greiner, et al. Legislation for smoke-free workplaces and health of bar workers in Ireland. *BMJ* (2005):331(7525):1117–22.

American Industrial Hygiene Association. *Recognition, Evaluation, and Control of Indoor Mold*. Prezant, B., D.M. Weekes, and J.D. Miller, eds. Fairfax, VA: American Industrial Hygiene Association, 2008.

American Society of Heating, Refrigerating, and Air-Conditioning Engineers Standard 62–2001. *Ventilation for Acceptable Indoor Air Quality*. Atlanta, GA: American Society of Heating, Refrigeration and Air-Conditioning Engineers, 2001.

Arbes, S.J. Jr., R.D. Cohn, M. Yin, et al. House dust mite allergen in US beds: Results from the First National Survey of Lead and Allergens in Housing. *J Allergy Clin Immunol* (2003):111(2):408–14.

Arbes, S.J. Jr., M. Sever, J. Archer, et al. Abatement of cockroach allergen (Bla g 1) in low-income, urban housing: A randomized controlled trial. *J Allergy Clin Immunol* (2003):112(2):339–45.

Arlian, L.G., D. Bernstein, I.L. Bernstein, et al. Prevalence of dust mites in the homes of people with asthma living in eight different geographic areas of the United States. *J Allergy Clin Immunol* (1992):90:292–300.

Arlian L.G., M.S. Morgan, and J.S. Neal. Dust mite allergens: ecology and distribution. *Curr All Asth Rep* (2002):2(5):401–11.

Ashengrau, A., A. Beiser, D. Bellinger, D. Copenhafer, and M. Weitzman. Residential lead-based paint hazard remediation and soil lead abatement: Their impact among children with mildly elevated blood lead levels. *Am J Public Health* (1997):87:1698–702.

Baker, M., A. McNicholas, N. Garrett, et al. Household crowding a major risk factor for epidemic meningococcal disease in Auckland children. *Pediatr Infect Dis J* (2000):19(10): 983–90.

Barn, P., T. Larson, M. Noullett, S. Kennedy, R. Copes, and M. Brauer. Infiltration of forest fire and residential wood smoke: An evaluation of air cleaner effectiveness. *J Expo Sci Environ Epidemiol* (2008):18(5):503–11.

Batterman, S., C. Godwin, and C.R. Jia. Long duration tests of room air filters in cigarette smokers' homes. *Environ Sci Technol* (2005):39(18):7260–8.

Bauman, K.E., R.L. Flewelling, and J. LaPrelle. Parental cigarette smoking and cognitive performance of children. *Health Psychol* (1991):10(4):282–8.

Berkowitz, G.S., J. Obel, E. Deych, et al. Exposure to indoor pesticides during pregnancy in a multiethnic, urban cohort. *Environ Health Perspect* (2003):111(1):79–84.

Bornschein, R.L., P.A. Succop, K.M. Kraft, et al. Exterior surface dust lead, interior house dust lead, and childhood lead exposure in an urban environment. In: Hemphill D.D., ed. *Trace Substances in Environmental Health-XX*. Proceedings of University of Missouri's 20th Annual Conference, June 1986. Columbia, MO: University of Missouri; 1987: 322–32.

Brodhead, B. Nationwide survey of RCP listed mitigation contractors. In: *1995 International Radon Symposium Proceedings*. Nashville, TN: American Association of Radiation Scientists and Technologists, 1995:III–5.1–5.14.

Burr, M.L., I.P. Matthews, R.A. Arthur, et al. Effects on patients with asthma of eradicating visible indoor mold: A randomised controlled trial. *Thorax* (2007):62(9):766–71.

Centers for Disease Control and Prevention. *Integrated Pest Management: Conducting Urban Rodent Surveys*. Atlanta, GA: US Department of Health and Human Services, 2006.

———. *Unintentional Non-Fire-Related Carbon Monoxide Exposures—United States, 2001–2003*. Atlanta, GA: U.S. Department of Health and Human Services, 2005.

Centers for Disease Control and Prevention and U.S. Department of Housing and Urban Development. *Healthy Housing Inspection Manual*. Atlanta, GA: Centers for Disease Control and Prevention and U.S. Department of Housing and Urban Development, 2007. Available at: http://www.healthyhomestraining.org/Practitioner/Essentials_Ref_Assess_Full_6-11-09.pdf.

———. *Healthy Housing Reference Manual*. Atlanta, GA: Centers for Disease Control and Prevention and U.S. Department of Housing and Urban Development, 2006. Available at: http://www.cdc.gov/nceh/publications/books/housing/housing.htm.

Chew, G., M.S. Perzanowski, S.M. Canfield, et al. Cockroach allergen levels and associations with cockroach-specific IgE. *J Allergy Clin Immunol* (2008):121(1):240–5.

Cohn, R.D. National prevalence and exposure risk for cockroach allergen in U.S. households. *Environ Health Perspect* (2006):114(4):522–6.

Consumer Product Safety Commission. *Ban of Lead-containing Paint and Certain Consumer Products Bearing Lead-containing Paint.* Bethesda, MD: Consumer Product Safety Commission, 1977. 16 CFR Part 1303.

Crane, J., I. Ellis, R. Siebers, D. Grimmet, S. Lewis, and P. Fitzharris. A pilot study of the effect of mechanical ventilation and heat exchange on house-dust mites and Der p 1 in New Zealand homes. *Allergy* (1998):53(8):755–62.

Dales, R., L. Liu, A.J. Wheeler, and N.L. Gilbert. Quality of indoor residential air and health. *Can Med Assoc J* (2008):179(2):147–52.

Darby, S. Radon in homes and risk of lung cancer: Collaborative analysis of individual data from 13 European case-control studies [see comment]. *BMJ* (2005):330(7485):223.

Diette, G.B., M.C. McCormack, N.N. Hansel, et al. Environmental issues in managing asthma. *Respir Care* (2008)53:602–15.

Dolkart, A. (n.d.). *The 1901 Tenement House Act.* Available at: http://www.tenement.org/features_dolkart.html. Accessed: June 16, 2010.

Eggleston, P.A., and L.K. Arruda. Ecology and elimination of cockroaches and allergens in the home. *J Allergy Clin Immunol* (2001):107(3 Suppl):S422–9.

Eggleston, P.A., A. Butz, C. Rand, et al. Home environmental intervention in inner-city asthma: A randomized controlled clinical trial. *Ann Allergy Asthma Immunol* (2005):95(6): 518–24.

Eskenazi, B., and L.S. Trupin. Passive and active maternal smoking during pregnancy, as measured by serum cotinine and postnatal smoke exposure. II. Effects on neurodevelopment at age 5 years. *Am J Epidemiol* (1995):42(9 Suppl):S19–29.

Eskenazi, B., L.G. Rosas, A.R. Marks, et al. Pesticide Toxicity and the Developing Brain. *Basic Clin Pharmacol Toxicol* (2008):102:228–36.

Evans, G.W., N.M. Wells, and A. Moch. Housing and mental health: A review of the evidence and a methodological and conceptual critique. *J Soc Issues* (2003):59:475–500.

Farfel, M.R., and J. J. Chisolm. Health and environmental outcomes of traditional and modified practices for abatement of residential lead-based paint. *Am J Public Health* (1990):80:1240–5.

Farfel, M.R., J.J. Chisolm, and C.A. Rohde. The longer-term effectiveness of residential lead paint abatement. *Environ Res* (1994):66:217–21.

Farrelly, M.C., J.M. Nonnemaker, R. Chou, A. Hyland, K.K. Peterson, and U.E. Bauer. Changes in hospitality workers' exposure to secondhand smoke following the implementation of New York's smoke-free law. *Tob Control* (2005):14(4):236–41.

Fergusson, D.M., L.J. Horwood, and M.T. Lynskey. Maternal smoking before and after pregnancy: Effects on behavioral outcomes in middle childhood. *Pediatrics* (1993):92(6):815–22.

Fong, G.T., A. Hyland, R. Borland, et al. Reductions in tobacco smoke pollution and increases in support for smoke-free public places following the implementation of comprehensive smoke-free workplace legislation in the Republic of Ireland: Findings from the ITC Ireland/UK Survey. *Tob Control* (2006):15:51–8.

Galea, S., N. Freudenberg, and D. Vlahov. Cities and population health. *Soc Sci Med* (2005):60(5):1017–33.

Groves-Kirkby, C.J., A.R. Denman, P.S. Phillips, et al. Radon mitigation in domestic properties and its health implications—a comparison between during-construction and postconstruction radon reduction. *Environ Int* (2006):32(4):435–43.

Gruchalla, R.S., J. Pongracic, M. Plaut, et al. Inner city asthma study: Relationships among sensitivity, allergen exposure, and asthma morbidity. *J Allergy Clin Immunol* (2005):115(3):478–85.

Haw, S.J., and L. Gruer. Changes in exposure of adult nonsmokers to secondhand smoke after implementation of smoke-free legislation in Scotland: National cross-sectional survey. *BMJ* (2007):335(7619):549. Epub 2007 Sep 9.

Huber, J., O. Ennemoser, and P. Schneider. Quality control of mitigation methods for unusually high indoor radon concentrations. *Health Phys* (2001):81(2):156–62.

Illi, S., E. von Mutius, S. Lau, B. Niggemann, C. Grüber, and U. Wahn; Multicentre Allergy Study (MAS) group. Perennial allergen sensitisation early in life and chronic asthma in children: A birth cohort study. *Lancet* (2006):368(9537):763–70.

Institute of Medicine. *Clearing the Air: Asthma and Indoor Air Exposures*. Washington, DC: National Academy Press, 2000.

——. *Damp Indoor Spaces and Health*. Washington, DC: National Academy Press, 2004. Jacobs, D.E., R.P. Clickner, J.Y. Zhou, et al. Prevalence of lead-based paint hazards in U.S. housing. *Environ Health Perspect* (2002):110(10):A599–606.

Jacobs, D.E., and A. Baeder. Housing interventions and health: A review of the evidence. National Center for Healthy Housing, Washington DC; 2009. Available at: http://www.nchh.org/LinkClick.aspx?fileticket=2lvaEDNBIdU%3d&tabid=229. Accessed July 16, 2010.

Jacobs, D.E., H. Mielke, and N. Pavur. The high cost of improper lead-based paint removal. *Environ Health Perspect* (2003):111:185–6.

Jones, R.L., D.M. Homa, P.A. Meyer, et al. Trends in blood lead level and blood lead testing among US children aged 1 to 5 years, 1988-2004. *Pediatrics* (2009):123:e376–85.

Kercsmar, C.M., D.G. Dearborn, M. Schluchter, et al. Reduction in asthma morbidity in children as a result of home remediation aimed at moisture sources. *Environ Health Perspect* (2006):114(10):1574–80.

Krewski, D., J.H. Lubin, J.M. Zielinski, et al. A combined analysis of North American case-control studies of residential radon and lung cancer. *J Toxicol Environ Health A* (2006):69(7):533–97.

Levin, R., M.J. Brown, M.E. Kashtock, et al. Lead exposure in US children, 2008: Implications for prevention. *Environ Health Perspect* (2008):116:1285–93.

Matsui, E.C, R.A. Wood, C. Rand, et al. Cockroach allergen exposure and sensitization in suburban middle-class children with asthma. *J Allergy Clin Immunol* (2003):112(1): 87–92.

Miller, D.M., F. Meek. Cost and efficacy comparison of integrated pest management strategies with monthly spray insecticide applications for German cockroach (Dictyoptera: Blattellidae) control in public housing. J Econ Entomol (2004):97:559–69.

National Center for Healthy Housing. *Evaluation of the HUD Lead Hazard Control Program.* Columbia, MD: National Center for Healthy Housing, 2004. Available at: http://www.nchh.org/Research/Archived-Research-Projects/HUD-Lead-Hazard-Control-Grant-Program.aspx.

National Center for Healthy Housing. Pediatric Environmental Home Assessment. Columbia, MD: National Center for Healthy Housing; 2009. Available at: http://www.healthy homestraining.org/Nurse/PEHA.htm.

——. *International Property Maintenance Code and Healthy Housing.* Columbia, MD: National Center for Healthy Housing, 2010. Available at: http://www.nchh.org/Policy/National-Policy/International-Property-Maintenance-Code.aspx.

National Research Council. *Measuring Lead Exposure in Infants, Children and Other Sensitive Populations.* Washington, DC: National Academy Press, 1993.

Nevin, R., D.E. Jacobs, M. Berg, and J. Cohen. Monetary benefits of preventing childhood lead poisoning with lead-safe window replacement. *Environ Res* (2008):106: 410–19.

Niven, R, A.M. Fletcher, A.C. Pickering, et al. Attempting to control mite allergens with mechanical ventilation and dehumidification in British houses. *J Allergy Clin Immunol* (1999):103(5 Pt 1):756–62.

Offerman, F.J. *Ventilation and Indoor Air Quality in New Homes. Indoor Environmental Engineering.* San Francisco, CA: California Air Resources Board; 2009. Available at: http://www.arb.ca.gov/research/apr/past/04-310main.pdf. 04-310.

Office of the Deputy Prime Minister, United Kingdom. *Preparation of the Housing Health and Safety Rating System*. London, England: Safe and Healthy Housing Research Unit, Warwick Law School, 2004.

Office of the Surgeon General. The Health Consequences of Involuntary Exposure to Tobacco Smoke: A Report of the Surgeon General. Washington DC; 2006. http://www.surgeongeneral.gov/library/secondhandsmoke/report/index.html

Pestka, J.J., I. Yike, D.G. Dearborn, and M.D. Ward. Stachybotrys chartarum, trichothecene mycotoxins, and damp building-related illness: New insights into a public health enigma. *Toxicol Sci* (2008):104(1):4–26.

Phipatanakul, W., P.A. Eggleston, E.C. Wright, and R.A. Wood. Mouse allergen. I. The prevalence of mouse allergen in inner-city homes. The National Cooperative Inner-City Asthma Study. *J Allergy Clin Immunol* (2000):106(6):1070–4.

Platts-Mills, T.A., and E.B. Mitchell. House dust mite avoidance. *Lancet* (1982):2(8311):1334.

Rauh, V.A., G.L. Chew, and R.S. Garfinkel. Deteriorated housing contributes to high cockroach allergen levels in inner-city households. *Environ Health Perspect* (2002):110(2):323–7.

Riis, J.A. *How the Other Half Lives: Studies among the Tenements of New York*. New York: Charles Scribner's Sons, 1890.

Salo, P.M., S.J. Arbes, P.W. Crockett, et al. Exposure to multiple indoor allergens in U.S. homes and its relationship to asthma. *J Allergy Clin Immunol* (2008):121:678–84.

Salo, P.M., M. Yin, S.J. Arbes, et al. Dustborne alternaria alternata antigens in U.S. homes: Results from the National Survey of Lead and Allergens. *J Allergy Clin Immunol* (2005):116(3):623–9.

Samet, J.M. Residential radon and lung cancer: End of the story? *J Toxicol Environ Health A* (2006):69(7):527–31.

Shaughnessy, R.J., and R.G. Sextro. What is an effective portable air cleaning device? A review. *J Occup Environ Hyg* (2006):3(4):169–81.

Stein, L. A study of respiratory tuberculosis in relation to housing conditions in Edinburgh; the pre-war period. *Br J Soc Med* (1950):4:143–69.

Title X. The Residential Lead Hazard Control Act of 1992. Public Law 102-550.

Tohn, E.R., S.L. Dixon, J.W. Wilson, W.A. Galke, and C.S. Clark. An evaluation of one-time professional cleaning in homes with lead-based paint hazards. *Appl Occup Environ Hyg* (2003):18(2):138–43.

Trasande, L., and G.D. Thurston. The role of air pollution in asthma and other pediatric morbidities. *J Allergy Clin Immunol* (2005):115(4):689–99.

Tuccillo, K., and F.B. Rauch. Evaluation and enforcement of radon mitigation system installations in New Jersey. In: *1994 International Radon Symposium*. Atlantic City, NJ: American Association of Radon Scientists and Technologists, 1994.

U.S. Department of Housing and Urban Development. *Guidelines for the Evaluation and Control of Lead-Based Paint Hazards in Housing*. HUD-1539. Washington, DC: U.S. Department of Housing and Urban Development, 1995. Available at: http://www.hud.gov/offices/lead/lbp/hudguidelines/index.cfm.

——. *Leading Our Nation to Healthier Homes: The Healthy Homes Strategic Plan*. Washington, DC: U.S. Department of Housing and Urban Development, 2009. Available at: http://www.hud.gov/offices/lead/library/hhi/DraftHHStratPlan_9.10.08.pdf.

U.S. Environmental Protection Agency. *Air Quality Criteria for Carbon Monoxide*. Washington, DC: U.S. EPA, National Center for Environmental Assessment, 2001.

——. *Assessment of Risks from Radon in Homes*. Washington, DC: Office of Air and Radiation, Indoor Environments Division, 2003.

——. *A Brief Guide to Mold, Moisture, and Your Home*. Washington, DC: Office of Air and Radiation Indoor Environments Division, 2002. (6609J) EPA 402-K-02-003.

——. *Consumer's Guide to Radon Reduction*. Washington, DC: U.S. EPA, 2010. Available at: http://www.epa.gov/radon/pubs/consguid.html. EPA 402K-10/002.

——. *Health Effects of Passive Smoking*. Washington, DC: U.S. EPA, Office of Research and Development, 1992.

——. *Pesticide Industry Sales and Usage: 2000 and 2001 Market Estimates*. Washington, DC: U.S. EPA, Office of Prevention, 2004.

——. *Radon Maps*. Washington, DC: U.S. EPA, 1993. Available at: http://www.epa.gov/radon/zonemap.html. Accessed June 16, 2010.

——. *Review of Studies Addressing Lead Abatement Effectiveness*. Updated edition. Washington, DC: U.S. EPA, 1998. Available at: http://www.epa.gov/lead/pubs/finalreport.pdf. EPA 747-B-98-001.

U.S. Public Health Service. APHA-CDC recommended housing maintenance and occupancy ordinance. Atlanta: US Department of Health and Human Services; 1975.

Wang, C.L., and G.W. Bennett. Comparative study of integrated pest management and baiting for German cockroach management in public housing. *J Econ Entomol* (2006):99(3):879–85.

Warner, J.A. J.M. Frederick, T.N. Bryant, et al. Mechanical ventilation and high-efficiency vacuum cleaning: A combined strategy of mite and mite allergen reduction in the control of mite-sensitive asthma. *J Allergy Clin Immunol* (2000):105(1):75–82.

Watson, W.A., T.L. Litovitz, G.C. Rodgers Jr., et al. 2002 annual report of the American Association of Poison Control Centers Toxic Exposure Surveillance System. *Am J Emerg Med* (2003):21(5):353–421.

Whyatt, R.M., D.E. Camann, P.L. Kinney, et al. Residential pesticide use during pregnancy among a cohort of urban minority women. *Environ Health Perspect* (2002):110(5):507–14.

Williams, G.M., M. O'Callaghan, J.M. Najman, et al. Maternal cigarette smoking and child psychiatric morbidity: A longitudinal study. *Pediatrics* (1998):102(1):e11.

Williams, M.K. An intervention to reduce residential insecticide exposure during pregnancy among an inner-city cohort. *Environ Health Perspect* (2006):114(11):1684–9.

Wilson, J., T. Pivetz, P. Ashley, et al. Evaluation of HUD-funded lead hazard control treatments at 6 years post-intervention. *Environ Res* (2006):102:237–48.

World Health Organization. *Report on the WHO Technical Meeting on Quantifying Disease from Inadequate Housing, Bonn, Germany, November 28–30, 2005.* Geneva, Switzerland: World Health Organization Regional Office for Europe.

——. *WHO Constitution* (1946). Available at: http://whqlibdoc.who.int/hist/official_records/constitution.pdf.

Principles of Healthy Housing: Safe

Angela Mickalide, PhD, CHES, and
Grant Baldwin, PhD, MPH

Safety is an integral component of a healthy home. According to a recent poll commissioned by the Home Safety Council, greater than 90% of parents and caregivers consider their home to be a safe haven (Mickalide 2006). Yet on average each year, unintentional injuries in the home result in approximately 20,000 deaths and 21 million medical visits (Runyan and Casteel 2004). Older adults have the highest rates of unintentional home injury deaths, as do males in every age group (Figure 3.1). Home-related injuries result in at least $222 billion in direct medical costs each year (Runyan and Casteel 2004). This chapter presents the epidemiology of the top five causes of unintentional home injury deaths (falls, poisoning, fires/burns, choking/suffocation, and drowning/submersion; Table 3.1), key concepts in disaster preparedness in the home, and prevention strategies for creating a safe home.

FALLS

Falls are a leading cause of unintentional injury morbidity and mortality in the home (Runyan, Casteel, et al. 2005; Runyan, Perkis, et al. 2005). Slightly more than 50% of all unintentional fall deaths and between 36% and 45% of all nonfatal injuries occur in the home (Runyan, Perkis, et al. 2005). Moreover, falls are the leading cause of emergency department visits for all home-related injuries (Runyan and Casteel 2004). Children and adults 65 years of age and older are at increased risk of a home-related fall (Runyan, Casteel, et al. 2005; Runyan, Perkis, et al.

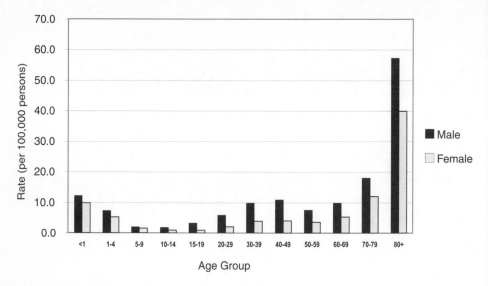

Source: With permission from the Home Safety Council (Runyan and Casteel 2004).

Figure 3.1—Unintentional home injury deaths. Average annual rate (per 100,000 persons), by age group and gender, United States, 1992–1999.

2005). The epidemiologic characteristics and recommended prevention strategies for each population are described in turn.

Children

Falls are the leading cause of nonfatal injuries for all children aged 0–19 years, not differentiating between those injuries happening in or out of the home (Borse et al. 2009). In addition, every day, approximately 8,000 children are treated in U.S. emergency departments for fall-related injuries, and falls account for 30% of all nonfatal injuries for children aged 0–19 years. However, there is variation by age group. For children less than 1 year of age, falls account for more than 50% of nonfatal injuries (Borse et al. 2009). An estimated 1.5 million children aged less than 15 years require medical attention from a home-related fall annually (Runyan et al. 2005). The percentage of fatal fall-related child injuries is small compared with other causes of child death. Approximately 1% of all fatal injuries for children aged 0–19 years are linked to falls (Borse et al. 2009). The risk of fall death is linked in part to the height of the fall and whether the fall occurs on an unforgiving surface (McDonald and Gielen 2006). Other factors include the velocity, the landing position, the mass of the individual, and whether the individual strikes an object during the fall.

TABLE 3.1 — UNINTENTIONAL HOME INJURY DEATHS: AVERAGE ANNUAL NUMBER, PERCENT-AGE, AND RATE (PER 100,000), ALL CAUSES, UNITED STATES, 1992–1999

Cause of Death	Number	Percentage	Rate
Fall	5,961	33.0	2.25
Poisoning	4,833	26.8	1.83
Fire/Burn	3,402	18.8	1.29
Choking/Suffocation	1,092	6.1	0.41
Drowning/Submersion	823	4.6	0.31
Firearm	590	3.3	0.22
Natural/Environmental	427	2.4	0.16
Struck By/Against	285	1.6	0.11
Miscellaneous	230	1.3	0.09
Unspecified	215	1.2	0.08
Machinery	127	0.7	0.05
Cut/Pierce	60	0.3	0.02
Overexertion	3	<0.1	<0.01
Motor Vehicle	0	0.0	0.00
Pedal Cyclist, Other	0	0.0	0.00
Pedestrian, Other	0	0.0	0.00
Transport, Other	0	0.0	0.00
TOTAL	18,048	100.0	6.83

Source: Data from the National Vital Statistics System, 1992–1999. With permission from the Home Safety Council.

Fatal and nonfatal falls disproportionately affect boys and children of low socioeconomic status and of a racial/ethnic minority (Borse et al. 2009; Fallat, Costich, and Pollack 2006; Khambalia et al. 2006; Shenassa, Stubbendick, and Brown 2004). Approximately 50% of the total number of disability-adjusted life years lost globally to falls occur in children aged less than 15 years (Peden, McGee, and Sharma 2002). Childhood falls represent a significant public health problem because of the associated morbidity.

There are characteristics of the child and the home environment that put children at greater risk of falling. A child's size, stage of development, and behavior all contribute to this increased risk (Mack, Gilchrist, and Ballesteros 2008; McDonald, Girasek, and Gielen 2005). Children have a higher center of gravity because a child's head is disproportionately larger than the rest of the body, making it easy for them to lose their balance. Children have a lack of fear, a limited ability to recognize hazards, and an attraction to potential hazards. As a result, a child may approach the top of stairs or climb on furniture without knowing the inherent risks.

There are a number of recommended prevention strategies to lower the risk of home-related childhood injuries from a fall. These can include redesigning or not using dangerous products, such as baby walkers and bunk beds; using home-safety devices, such as guards on windows that are above ground level, stair gates, and guard rails; and using enhanced caregiver supervision (Kendrick et al. 2008; Kendrick et al. 2008; McDonald, Girasek, and Gielen 2005). More energy-absorbing flooring and playground surfaces, rounded counter tops, and padded furniture guards are important secondary prevention strategies (Khambalia et al. 2006; McDonald, Girasek, and Gielen 2005).

Older Adults

Each year, approximately one third of older adults fall, and the risk of falling and home-related fall death increases dramatically with age (Centers for Disease Control and Prevention [CDC] 2008a; Runyan et al. 2005). In 2005, approximately 16,000 persons 65 years of age and older died as a result of a fall, including all locations of a fall (CDC 2006a). Between 10% and 16% of older adults fell in a 3-month period in 2006, and 1.8 million people who fell visited a health care provider or were limited in their daily activity (Boyd and Stevens 2009; CDC 2006a). A greater number of older men die and a greater number of older women are likely to sustain an injury in a home-related fall (Runyan et al. 2005; Runyan et al. 2005).

After an older adult falls, he or she is at increased risk of falling again and may develop a fear of falling, resulting in loss of independence, social isolation, depression, and mobility restriction (Boyd and Stevens 2009; Scheffer et al. 2008). More than one third or 12.8 million older adults are moderately or very afraid of falling (Boyd and Stevens 2009).

The cost of falls in older adults is substantial. In 2000, the direct medical costs totaled $0.2 billion for fatal falls and $19 billion for nonfatal falls (Stevens et al. 2006). Although these costs are not specific to falls occurring in the home, the costs associated with home-related falls are likely significant given their incidence and the percentage of time older adults spend at home.

The role home hazards play in increasing the risk of falling is not straightforward, especially among older adults (Lord, Menz, and Sherrington 2006). Most older adult home-related falls result from a complicated interaction between home hazards and individual susceptibility linked to muscle weakness, gait and balance problems, poor vision, and multiple medication use (Rubenstein 2006; Stevens and Sogolow 2005). Making home modifications, such as installing handrails on stairs, placing grab bars in bathrooms, and improving lighting *without* attending to other risk factors will not reduce the risk of falling for older adults (Lord, Menz, and Sherrington 2006). That said, reducing home hazards is an important component of a multifaceted intervention, especially among adults 75 years of age and older and persons with mobility limitation (Lord, Menz, and Sherrington 2006). The most effective and cost-saving interventions include comprehensive risk factor assessment linked to targeted interventions, including exercise (balance, strength, flexibility, and endurance training), medication management, vision correction, and home modification (Rubenstein 2006; Rubenstein and Josephson 2006; Rubenstein, Stevens, and Scott 2007; Stevens and Sogolow 2008).

POISONING

Poisonings are the second leading cause of home injury death in the United States, resulting in approximately 5,000 deaths per year (Runyan and Casteel 2004). Although most public education campaigns have targeted poisoning prevention among children, adults aged 20–59 years have the highest poisoning death rates at home. At particular risk are adults aged 40–49 years, followed by those aged 30–39 years (Runyan and Casteel 2004).

Many of these deaths are due to misuse of prescription medication, which has increased dramatically in the United States. In 2005, approximately 30,000 people died of an unintended or undetermined-intent poisoning in the United States—more than a 70% increase compared with same-type deaths recorded in 1999 (Paulozzi, Ballesteros, and Stevens 2006). Prescription pain medications, such as methadone, oxycodone, hydrocodone, morphine, and fentanyl, are largely responsible for the alarming increase in drug poisoning death rates. In addition to recorded deaths from unintentional poisoning, the CDC reports that in 2006 more than 700,000 people in America sought emergency medical attention as a result of misuse of medication, and a quarter of these individuals required hospitalization (CDC 2009).

In contrast with high poisoning fatality rates among adults, children younger than 5 years of age have the highest nonfatal poisoning rates because of exposure to cosmetics/personal care products, household cleaners, and medications (Runyan and Casteel 2004). In 2007, more than half of all poison exposures (51.2%) reported to poison control centers occurred among children younger than 6 years of age (Bronstein et al. 2008).

Carbon monoxide (CO) is an odorless, colorless, and tasteless poisonous gas that is emitted from fossil-fuel burning sources, such as stoves, heaters, and motor vehicles. CO results from the incomplete burning of coal, oil, kerosene, propane, wood, charcoal, and natural gas (U.S. Consumer Product Safety Commission 2009). Each year in the United States, approximately 500 people die and 20,000 people visit emergency departments for CO exposure, although not all of them occur in the home environment (CDC 2008).

Recommended strategies for poisoning prevention include locking potentially poisonous products out of reach of children and teenagers, using child-resistant packaging, installing CO detectors in sleeping areas and basements, and posting the national toll-free poison control number (1-800-222-1222) on or near telephones. A person should also be advised to follow directions on the label when he or she gives or takes medicines and to read all warning labels because some medicines cannot be taken safely when other medicines or alcohol is consumed. In addition, a person should turn on a light when giving or taking medicines at night so that he or she knows that the dosage is correct. All medicines should be kept in their original bottles or containers. Prescription drugs should never be shared or sold. Opioid pain medications, such as methadone, hydrocodone, and oxycodone, should be kept in a safe place that can be reached only by people who take or administer them. Monitor the use of medicines prescribed for children and teenagers, such as medicines for attention deficit disorder or attention deficit hyperactivity disorder. People should dispose of unused, unneeded, or expired prescription drugs by following the federal guidelines for how to do this without harming others or the environment.

FIRE AND BURNS

Fire and burn injuries are the third leading cause of home injury death, resulting in approximately 3,400 fatalities per year (Runyan and Casteel 2004). Adults aged 70 years and older have the highest death rates, followed by children aged less than 5 years. These two populations are at excess risk because they may react more slowly in fires because of limited mobility, and they spend more time in the home compared with other age groups. Males have higher death rates than females across the life span. In addition, more than 261,000 nonfatal fire and burn injuries requiring medical attention occur on average each year in homes across America (Runyan and Casteel 2004).

Recommended strategies to reduce fire- and burn-related deaths and injuries at home include storing matches and lighters locked out of reach of children, using back burners while cooking, setting water heaters to 120°F, using temperature-controlled mixer faucets, installing and maintaining working smoke alarms on every level of the home and in bedrooms and sleeping areas, creating and practicing a home escape plan, and installing automatic residential fire sprinklers in new and existing homes (Warda and Ballesteros 2007). Installed, working smoke alarms have been shown to lower the fire death rate by 40%–50% compared with homes without them (Ahrens 2004). Other interventions are promising or in need of formative research (DiGuiseppi et al., in press).

AIRWAY OBSTRUCTION

Airway obstruction includes suffocation—when an object covers one's nose or mouth; strangulation—when something compresses one's neck, making it difficult to breath; and choking—when a small object gets lodged in one's throat or windpipe (McDonald, Girasek, and Gielen 2005).

In 2006, approximately 6,000 people died of unintentional choking or suffocation (CDC 2006b). Children aged less than 1 year and older adults aged more than 65 years are at greatest risk (CDC 2006b). For children aged less than 1 year, two-thirds of injury deaths were due to suffocation, and the rate was more than 16 times greater than the rate for children aged 1–19 years (Borse et al. 2009). For children aged less than 14 years, airway obstruction is the second most lethal form of child injury: There is 1 death for every 14 visits to the emergency department (Ballesteros et al. 2003). Across all ages, males have higher rates of choking or suffocation death than do females (Borse et al. 2009; Runyan and Casteel 2004). The mechanism and circumstances of suffocation and choking are age specific (Vilke et al. 2004). Children have an insatiable curiosity and urge to explore. Children also mouth objects as a way to explore. Children have an inability to chew and swallow certain foods. This can expose them to choking and suffocation hazards (Runyan and Casteel 2004).

Choking and suffocation injuries are the fourth leading cause of home-related unintentional injury death in the United States (Runyan and Casteel 2004). Approximately 25% of all choking and suffocation deaths occur at home, and this may underrepresent the nature of the problem given that the location of these fatalities are not known in 60% of the cases (Runyan and Casteel 2004). Overall, suffocations in the home cost the United States more than $3 billion annually (Zaloshnja et al. 2005).

For every choking-related death, there are approximately 100 visits to emergency departments (CDC 2002). A total of 60% of nonfatal choking episodes treated in emergency departments are associated with food items such as hot dogs, hard candies, nuts, grapes, and popcorn; 31% involve non-food objects such as coins, marbles, and balloons; and the remaining 9% are unknown for children less than 14 years old (CDC 2002). Approximately 70% of all nonfatal unintentional choking and suffocation injuries occur at home (Runyan and Casteel 2004). More than 37,000 emergency department visits are linked to obstructed airway injuries in the home (Runyan and Casteel 2004).

Cribs, beds, and bedding are involved in approximately 50% of infant suffocations, and African American male infants less than 4 months old are at elevated risk (Drago and Dannenberg 1999; Shapiro-Mendoza et al. 2009). Infants suffocate when their faces become buried in a mattress, pillow, or other soft bedding or when a bed-sharing caregiver rolls over on them (McDonald, Girasek, and Gielen 2005).

The most common items causing childhood strangulation include clothing drawstrings, ribbons, necklaces, pacifier strings, window blind/drapery cords, cribs, bunk beds, playground equipment, or other furniture with improperly spaced slats (McDonald, Girasek, and Gielen 2005; Nixon et al. 1995). The U.S. Consumer Product Safety Commission, a federal agency working to ensure the safety of consumer products, has issued warnings on items that pose a choking or suffocation hazard, including toys with small parts, bedding, strings and cords, toy chests, and accordion-style baby gates (McDonald, Girasek, and Gielen 2005).

There are a number of recommended strategies to prevent airway obstruction. The most prominent prevention strategy is focused on product regulation (Tarrago 2000). Additional strategies focus on the importance of supervising young children at all times; not feeding young children foods or providing access to small objects that are known choking hazards; adhering to age-related product warnings on toys and instructions on child restraints and other household products; and educating caregivers on the risks of co-sleeping or placing infants to sleep on adult beds and sofas and chairs (IMPACT 2005). Caregivers need to be trained in infant/child cardiopulmonary resuscitation and the Heimlich maneuver (IMPACT 2005; McDonald, Girasek, and Gielen 2005).

DROWNING/SUBMERSION

Among all age groups in the United States, children have the highest rates of drowning, especially children 1–4 years of age, for whom drowning is the leading cause of injury death (Borse et al. 2009, Table 3; CDC 2004). A small child can drown in a few centimeters of water in a bathtub or bucket (Brenner et al. 2001). Approximately 7,000 U.S. children 0–19 years of age drowned between 2000 and

2005, and 27% of these deaths were among children 1–4 years of age (Borse et al. 2009). Because drowning disproportionately affects youth, drowning is the third leading cause of years of potential life lost among unintentional injuries in youth (Brenner 2003).

For every 1 drowning, there are 4 cases of nonfatal drowning, which is surviving for at least 24 hours after suffocation from submersion in water (Brenner 2003; Fields 1992; Wintemute 1990). Males are 2–10 times more likely to drown than females, and African Americans, American Indians, and Asian Americans have higher death rates than Whites (Brenner et al. 2001; CDC 2004; Quan, Bennett, and Branche 2007). In the United States, drowning rates are highest in the southeast, west, and Alaska (Borse et al. 2009). Among children less than 15 years of age, approximately two thirds of all drowning incidents occur in the summer months (May to August), and drownings disproportionately occur on weekends (Brenner 2003; Kane, Mickalide, and Paul 2001). In 2000, the total lifetime cost of fatal and nonfatal drowning among children less than 4 years of age was $1.8 billion (Finkelstein, Corso, and Miller 2006).

Drowning is the fifth leading cause of unintentional home injury death. Although nonfatal drowning is not a leading cause of home injury, approximately 10,000 nonfatal drownings occur in the home each year, requiring medical care or emergency department treatment, and result in days away from work or school. Slightly more than 20% of all drownings occur in the home or surrounding areas (Runyan and Casteel 2004).

The site of drownings varies by age group. Children less than 1 year old are most likely to drown in bathtubs (55% of all deaths). Swimming pools are the most likely location of drowning for children 1–4 years of age (56% of all deaths). Children 5–19 years of age are most likely to die in fresh bodies of water, such as rivers and lakes (63% of all deaths) (Brenner et al. 2001).

In a recent survey, more than 90% of parents with children aged less than 14 years report that their children swim. However, only one third of parents recognize drowning as the second leading cause of unintentional injury death for their children (Quaraishi et al. 2006).

Recommended strategies to reduce the risk of drowning or nonfatal drowning in the home are dependent on the age of the person and circumstances of the event and should include a combination of environmental and behavioral interventions (Brenner 2003; Quan and Cummings 2003). Drowning-prevention strategies deemed to be effective include constant adult supervision of infants in bathtubs and all children in other swimming areas, installation of four-sided pool fencing with self-closing and self-latching gates, and use of personal flotation devices (Brenner 2003; Quan et al. 2007; Simon, Tamura, and Colton 2003). Proper pool fencing alone can reduce the risk of drowning by more than 50% (Thompson and Rivara 2000). Formal swimming lessons are strongly associated with a lower risk of drowning for children 1–4 years of age, and these lessons may offer a protective effect for older children and adolescents (Brenner et al. 2009). That said, swimming lessons should not take the place of the other primary prevention strategies listed earlier, and the best prevention strategy is to use all known effective interventions simultaneously (Quan et al. 2007; Rivara 2009).

In the event of a nonfatal drowning, parents and caregivers are advised to take training in basic lifesaving skills because resuscitation, if initiated immediately, results in significantly better neurologic and other health outcomes (Kyriacou et al. 1994; Quan and Kinder 1992). Other promising strategies that could complement the prevention strategies listed earlier for home drowning prevention are pool/door alarms—audible devices designed to alert caregivers when a door leading to a swimming pool area is opened—and drain covers and anti-entrapment devices (Brenner 2003; Quan et al. 2007; Quaraishi et al. 2006).

DISASTER PREPAREDNESS

Floods, tornadoes, heat waves, earthquakes, droughts, landslides, and other natural disasters wreak havoc on individuals, families, and communities. Each year in the United States, hundreds of people die and thousands more are injured in disasters, such as Hurricane Katrina and the record-breaking blizzard of 2010. Acts of terrorism, such as the September 11, 2001, World Trade Center tragedy, disrupt lives emotionally, mentally, and physically. Yet according to the results of several public opinion polls, many people in America think that "it is not going to happen to me" (Home Safety Council 2010; Operation Hope 2010) and do not complete common preparedness measures (Diekman et al. 2007). There are two necessary steps to prepare for disasters. The first is creating a communications plan for reaching family members, out-of-state relatives and friends, emergency services personnel, health care providers, and other key contacts. The second is creating "ready-to-stay" and "ready-to-go" kits to enhance survival. Such kits should include flashlights, fresh batteries, nonperishable food, medicines, a first aid kit, personal hygiene supplies, extra clothing and blankets, copies of important documents, a battery-operated or hand-crank radio, and one gallon of water per person per day for at least three days, among other items. Several national organizations such as the American Red Cross and the Home Safety Council, umbrella groups such as the Coalition of Organizations for Disaster Education (2007), and governmental entities such as the Federal Emergency Management Agency and the CDC provide additional

TABLE 3.2—EASY TO READ HOME INJURY CHECKLISTS

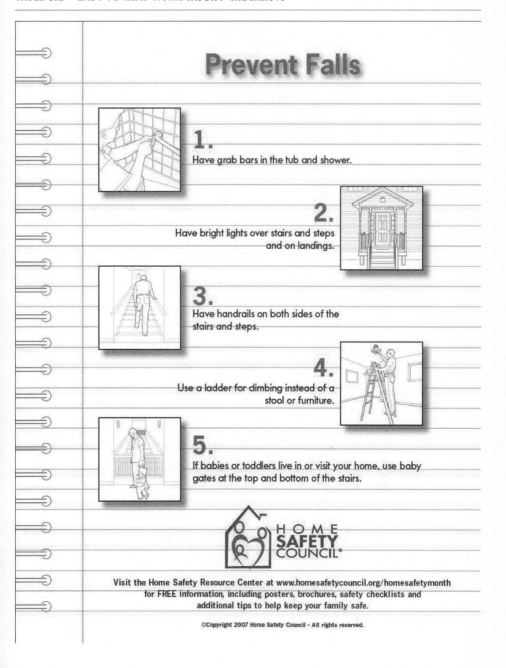

Prevent Falls

1.
Have grab bars in the tub and shower.

2.
Have bright lights over stairs and steps and on landings.

3.
Have handrails on both sides of the stairs and steps.

4.
Use a ladder for climbing instead of a stool or furniture.

5.
If babies or toddlers live in or visit your home, use baby gates at the top and bottom of the stairs.

HOME SAFETY COUNCIL®

Visit the Home Safety Resource Center at www.homesafetycouncil.org/homesafetymonth for FREE information, including posters, brochures, safety checklists and additional tips to help keep your family safe.

TABLE 3.2 — (CONTINUED)

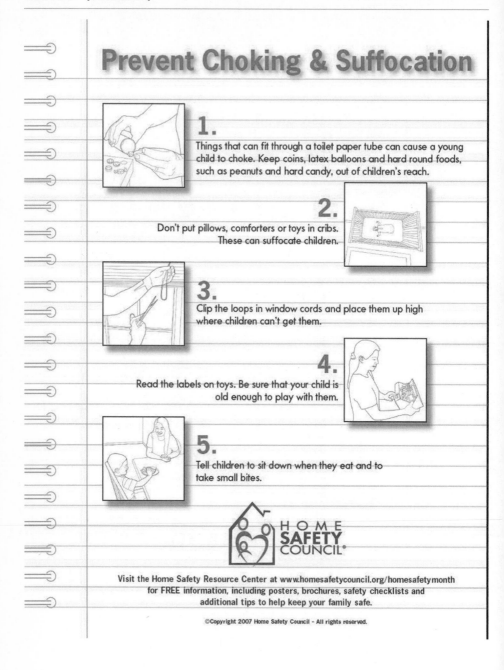

Prevent Choking & Suffocation

1.
Things that can fit through a toilet paper tube can cause a young child to choke. Keep coins, latex balloons and hard round foods, such as peanuts and hard candy, out of children's reach.

2.
Don't put pillows, comforters or toys in cribs. These can suffocate children.

3.
Clip the loops in window cords and place them up high where children can't get them.

4.
Read the labels on toys. Be sure that your child is old enough to play with them.

5.
Tell children to sit down when they eat and to take small bites.

HOME
SAFETY
COUNCIL®

Visit the Home Safety Resource Center at www.homesafetycouncil.org/homesafetymonth for FREE information, including posters, brochures, safety checklists and additional tips to help keep your family safe.

TABLE 3.2 — (CONTINUED)

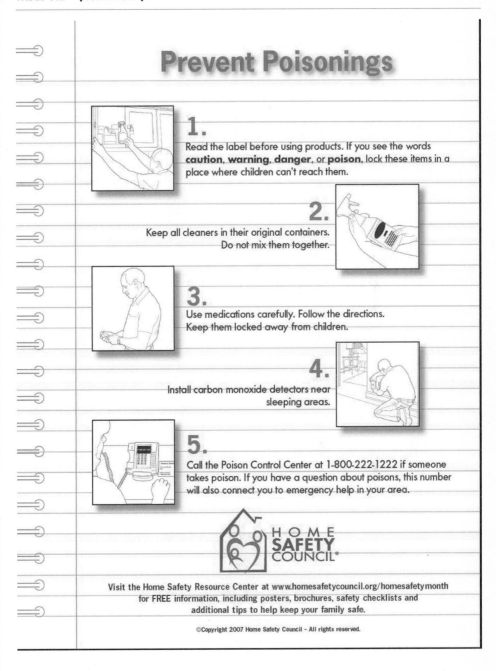

Prevent Poisonings

1.
Read the label before using products. If you see the words **caution, warning, danger,** or **poison,** lock these items in a place where children can't reach them.

2.
Keep all cleaners in their original containers. Do not mix them together.

3.
Use medications carefully. Follow the directions. Keep them locked away from children.

4.
Install carbon monoxide detectors near sleeping areas.

5.
Call the Poison Control Center at 1-800-222-1222 if someone takes poison. If you have a question about poisons, this number will also connect you to emergency help in your area.

HOME
SAFETY
COUNCIL®

Visit the Home Safety Resource Center at www.homesafetycouncil.org/homesafetymonth for FREE information, including posters, brochures, safety checklists and additional tips to help keep your family safe.

TABLE 3.2 — (CONTINUED)

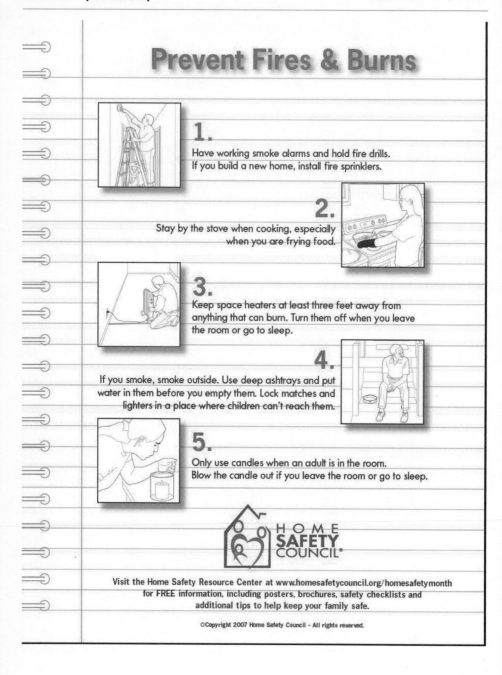

Prevent Fires & Burns

1. Have working smoke alarms and hold fire drills. If you build a new home, install fire sprinklers.

2. Stay by the stove when cooking, especially when you are frying food.

3. Keep space heaters at least three feet away from anything that can burn. Turn them off when you leave the room or go to sleep.

4. If you smoke, smoke outside. Use deep ashtrays and put water in them before you empty them. Lock matches and lighters in a place where children can't reach them.

5. Only use candles when an adult is in the room. Blow the candle out if you leave the room or go to sleep.

HOME
SAFETY
COUNCIL®

Visit the Home Safety Resource Center at www.homesafetycouncil.org/homesafetymonth for FREE information, including posters, brochures, safety checklists and additional tips to help keep your family safe.

TABLE 3.2—(CONTINUED)

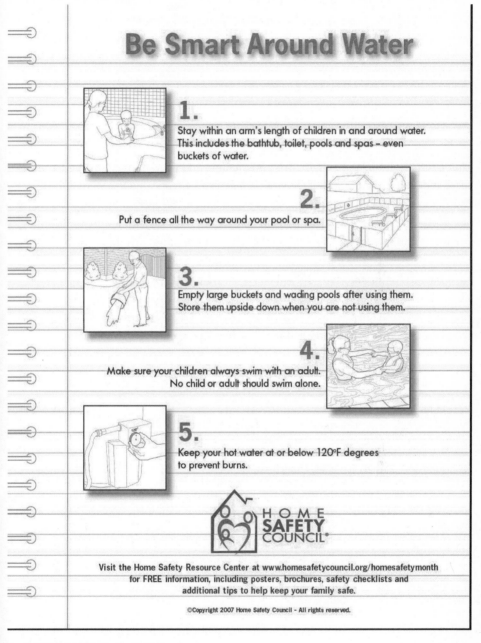

Be Smart Around Water

1. Stay within an arm's length of children in and around water. This includes the bathtub, toilet, pools and spas – even buckets of water.

2. Put a fence all the way around your pool or spa.

3. Empty large buckets and wading pools after using them. Store them upside down when you are not using them.

4. Make sure your children always swim with an adult. No child or adult should swim alone.

5. Keep your hot water at or below 120°F degrees to prevent burns.

HOME
SAFETY
COUNCIL®

Visit the Home Safety Resource Center at www.homesafetycouncil.org/homesafetymonth for FREE information, including posters, brochures, safety checklists and additional tips to help keep your family safe.

Source: With permission from the Home Safety Council.

guidance for disaster preparedness. Because both natural and human-caused disasters can occur in the blink of an eye in any community, it is essential for everyone to make the effort to be prepared (Trust for America's Health 2009) and to help others prepare, especially children (National Commission on Children and Disasters 2010), the elderly, and people with disabilities (National Organization on Disability 2009).

CONCLUSION

Unintentional home injuries are both predictable and preventable. Through a multi-faceted approach combining behavioral change, adequate supervision of children, installation and maintenance of safety devices, and adherence to building codes and safety regulations and legislation, all people can live in safer homes. In addition, by preparing for natural disasters or acts of terrorism, families can more easily shelter-in-place or evacuate to a better environment, depending on the circumstances. Refer to Table 3.2 for simple steps individuals and families can take to ensure that their abode is truly a safe haven. Safety is one of the key principles of healthy housing, and time, money, and energy must be invested to reduce the 55 deaths and the approximately 57,500 medically attended injuries that occur in the home every day.

REFERENCES
Ahrens, M. *U.S. Experience with Smoke Alarms and Other Fire Alarms.* Quincy, MA: National Fire Protection Association, 2004.

Ballesteros, M.F., R.A. Schieber, J. Gilchrist, P. Holmgreen, and J.L. Annest. Differential ranking of causes of fatal versus non-fatal injuries among US children. *Inj Prev* 2003:9(2):173–6.

Borse, N.N., J. Gilchrist, A.M. Dellinger, R.A. Rudd, M.F. Ballesteros, and D.A. Sleet. CDC *Childhood Injury Report: Patterns of Unintentional Injuries among 0–19 Year Olds in the United States, 2000–2006.* Atlanta, GA: Centers for Disease Control and Prevention, National Center for Injury Prevention and Control, 2009.

Boyd, R., and J. Stevens. Falls and fear of falling: Burden, beliefs and behaviours. *Age Ageing* 2009:38:423–8. Epub 2009 May 6.

Brenner, R.A. Prevention of drowning in infants, children, and adolescents. *Pediatrics* 2003:112(2):440–5.

Brenner, R.A., G.S. Taneja, D.L. Haynie, et al. Association between swimming lessons and drowning in childhood: A case-control study. *Arch Pediatr Adolesc Med* 2009:163(3):203–10.

Brenner, R.A., A.C. Trumble, G.S. Smith, E.P. Kessler, and M.D. Overpeck. Where children drown, United States, 1995. *Pediatrics* 2001:108(1):85–9.

Bronstein, A.C., D.A. Spyker, L.R. Cantilena, et al. 2007 Annual Report of the American Association of Poison Control Centers' National Poison Data System (NPDS): 25th Annual Report. *Clin Toxicol (Phila)* 2008:46:927–1057.

Centers for Disease Control and Prevention. Fatalities and injuries from falls among older adults—United States, 1993–2003 and 2001–2005. *MMWR Morb Mortal Wkly Rep* 2006a:55(45):1221–4.

——. Nonfatal and fatal drownings in recreational water settings—United States, 2001–2002. *MMWR Morb Mortal Wkly Rep* 2004:53(21):447–52.

——. Nonfatal choking-related episodes among children—United States, 2001. *MMWR Morb Mortal Wkly Rep* 2002:51(42):945–8.

——. *Poisoning in the United States: Fact Sheet* (2010). Available at: http://www.cdc.gov/HomeandRecreationalSafety/Poisoning/poisoning-factsheet.htm. Accessed August 5, 2010.

——. *The Quiet Killer* [transcript] (2008). Available at: http://www.cdc.gov/CDCTV/Quiet Killer/Transcripts/QuietKiller.pdf. Accessed August 5, 2010.

——. Self-reported falls and fall-related injuries among persons aged > or =65 years—United States, 2006. *MMWR Morb Mortal Wkly Rep* 2008a:57(9):225–9.

——. *Web-based Injury Statistics Query and Reporting System* (2006b). Available at: www.cdc.gov/ncipc/wisqars. Accessed June 17, 2009.

Coalition of Organizations for Disaster Education. *Talking About Disasters: A Guide to Standard Messages.* Washington, DC: American Red Cross, 2007.

Diekman, S.T., S.P. Kearney, M.E. O'Neil, and K.A. Mack. Qualitative study of homeowners' emergency preparedness: Experiences, perceptions, and practices. *Prehosp Disaster Med* 2007:22(6):494–501.

DiGuiseppi, C., D. Jacobs, and K. Phelan, et al. Housing interventions and control of injury-related structural deficiencies: A review of the evidence. *J Public Health Manage Pract.* In press.

Drago, D.A., and A.L. Dannenberg. Infant mechanical suffocation deaths in the United States, 1980–1997. *Pediatrics* 1999:103(5):e59.

Fallat, M.E., J. Costich, and A. Pollack. The impact of disparities in pediatric trauma on injury-prevention initiatives. *J Trauma* 2006:60(2):452–4.

Fields, A.I. Near-drowning in the pediatric population. *Crit Care Clin* 1992:8(1):113–29.

Finkelstein, E., P.S. Corso, and T.R. Miller. *The Incidence and Economic Burden of Injuries in the United States.* New York: Oxford University Press, 2006.

Home Safety Council. *Disaster Preparedness Survey of Mothers and their Children* (2010). Available at: http://homesafetycouncil.org/aboutus/research /re_survey_w002.asp. Accessed July 5, 2010.

IMPACT. *A Review of Best Practices—Preventing Suffocation and Choking Injuries in Manitoba.* Winnipeg, Manitoba, Canada: Manitoba Health, 2005.

Kane, B.E., A.D. Mickalide, and H.A. Paul. *Trauma Season: A National Study of the Seasonality of Unintentional Childhood Injury.* Washington, DC: National SAFE KIDS Campaign, 2001.

Kendrick, D., J. Barlow, A. Hampshire, S. Stewart-Brown, and L. Polnay. Parenting interventions and the prevention of unintentional injuries in childhood: Systematic review and meta-analysis. *Child Care Health Dev* 2008:34(5):682–95.

Kendrick, D., M.C. Watson, C.A. Mulvaney, et al. Preventing childhood falls at home: Meta-analysis and meta-regression. *Am J Prev Med* 2008:35(4):370–9.

Khambalia, A., P. Joshi, M. Brussoni, P. Raina, B. Morrongiello, and C. Macarthur. Risk factors for unintentional injuries due to falls in children aged 0–6 years: A systematic review. *Inj Prev* 2006:12(6):378–81.

Kyriacou, D.N., E.L. Arcinue, C. Peek, and J.F. Kraus. Effect of immediate resuscitation on children with submersion injury. *Pediatrics* 1994:94(2 Pt 1):137–42.

Lord, S.R., H.B. Menz, and C. Sherrington. Home environment risk factors for falls in older people and the efficacy of home modifications. *Age Ageing* 2006:35(Suppl 2):ii55–9.

Mack, K.A., J. Gilchrist, and M.F. Ballesteros. Injuries among infants treated in emergency departments, United States, 2001–2004. *Pediatrics* 2008:121(5):930–7.

McDonald, E., and A.C. Gielen. House fires and other unintentional home injuries. In: Gielen, A.C., D.A. Sleet, and R.J. DiClemente, eds. *Injury and Violence Prevention: Behavioral Science Theories, Methods and Applications.* San Francisco: Jossey-Bass, 2006: pp. 274–96.

McDonald, E., D.C. Girasek, and A.C. Gielen. Home injuries. In: DeSafey, Liller K., ed. *Injury Prevention for Children and Adolescents: Research, Practice and Advocacy.* Washington, DC: American Public Health Association, 2005: pp. 123–62.

Mickalide, A.D. *Safe Haven: A National Survey of Parents' Home Safety Perceptions and Actions.* Washington, DC: Home Safety Council, 2006.

National Commission on Children and Disasters. *Interim Report* (2010). Available at: http://www.childrenanddisasters.acf.hhs.gov. Accessed July 5, 2010.

National Organization on Disability. *Functional Needs of People with Disabilities: A Guide for Emergency Managers, Planners, and Responders.* Washington, DC: National Organization on Disability, 2009.

Nixon, J.W., A.M. Kemp, S. Levene, and J.R. Sibert. Suffocation, choking, and strangulation in childhood in England and Wales: Epidemiology and prevention. *Arch Dis Child* 1995:72(1):6–10.

Operation Hope. *Few Americans Prepared for Disaster* (2010). Available at: http://www. consumeraffairs.com/news04/2006/01/disaster_planning.html. Accessed July 5, 2010.

Paulozzi, L.P., M.F. Ballesteros, and J.A. Stevens. Recent trends in mortality from unintentional injury in the United States. *J Safety Res* 2006:37:277–83.

Peden, M., K. McGee, and G. Sharma. *The Injury Chart Book: A Graphical Overview of the Global Burden of Injuries*. Geneva: World Health Organization, 2002.

Quan, L., E.E. Bennett, and C.M. Branche. Interventions to prevent drowning. In: Doll, L.S., S.E. Bonzo, J.A. Mercy, D.A. Sleet, eds. *Handbook of Injury and Violence Prevention*. New York: Springer, 2007: pp. 81–96.

Quan, L., and P. Cummings. Characteristics of drowning by different age groups. *Inj Prev* 2003:9(2):163–8.

Quan, L., and D. Kinder. Pediatric submersions: Prehospital predictors of outcome. *Pediatrics* 1992:90(6):909–13.

Quaraishi, A.Y., S. Morton, B.E. Cody, and R. Wilcox. *Pool and Spa Drowning: A National Study of Drain Entrapment and Pool Safety Measures*. Washington, DC: Safe Kids Worldwide, 2006.

Rivara, F.P. Prevention of drowning: The time is now. *Arch Pediatr Adolesc Med* 2009:163(3):277–8.

Rubenstein, L.Z. Falls in older people: Epidemiology, risk factors and strategies for prevention. *Age Ageing* 2006:35(Suppl 2):ii37–41.

Rubenstein, L.Z., and K.R. Josephson. Falls and their prevention in elderly people: What does the evidence show? *Med Clin North Am* 2006:90(5):807–24.

Rubenstein, L.Z., J.A. Stevens, and V. Scott. Interventions to prevent falls among older adults. In: Doll, L.S., S.E. Bonzo, J.A. Mercy, and D.A. Sleet, eds. *Handbook of Injury and Violence Prevention*. New York: Springer, 2007: pp 37–53.

Runyan, C.W., and C. Casteel. *The State of Home Safety in America: Facts about Unintentional Injuries in the Home*. Washington, DC: Home Safety Council, 2004.

Runyan, C.W., C. Casteel, D. Perkis, et al. Unintentional injuries in the home in the United States Part I: Mortality. *Am J Prev Med* 2005:28(1):73–9.

Runyan, C.W., D. Perkis, S.W. Marshall, et al. Unintentional injuries in the home in the United States Part II: Morbidity. *Am J Prev Med* 2005:28(1):80–7.

Scheffer, A.C., M.J. Schuurmans, N. van Dijk, T. van der Hooft, and S.E. de Rooij. Fear of falling: Measurement strategy, prevalence, risk factors and consequences among older persons. *Age Ageing* 2008:37(1):19–24.

Shapiro-Mendoza, C.K., M. Kimball, K.M. Tomashek, R.N. Anderson, and S. Blanding, S. US infant mortality trends attributable to accidental suffocation and strangulation in bed from 1984 through 2004: Are rates increasing? *Pediatrics* 2009:123(2):533–9.

Shenassa, E.D., A. Stubbendick, and M.J. Brown. Social disparities in housing and related pediatric injury: A multilevel study. *Am J Public Health* 2004:94(4):633–9.

Simon, H.K., T. Tamura, and K. Colton. Reported level of supervision of young children while in the bathtub. *Ambul Pediatr* 2003:3(2):106–8.

Stevens, J.A., P.S. Corso, E.A. Finkelstein, and T.R. Miller. The costs of fatal and non-fatal falls among older adults. *Inj Prev* 2006:12(5):290–5.

Stevens, J.A., and E.D. Sogolow. Gender differences for non-fatal unintentional fall related injuries among older adults. *Inj Prev* 2005:11(2):115–9.

———. *Preventing Falls: What Works. A CDC Compendium of Effective Community-based Interventions from Around the World.* Atlanta, GA: Centers for Disease Control and Prevention, National Center for Injury Prevention and Control, 2008.

Tarrago, S.B. Prevention of choking, strangulation, and suffocation in childhood. *WMJ* 2000:99(9):42–6.

Thompson, D.C., and F.P. Rivara. Pool fencing for preventing drowning in children. *Cochrane Database Syst Rev* 2000:(2):CD001047.

Trust for America's Health. *Ready or Not? Protecting the Public's Health from Diseases, Disasters, and Bioterrorism.* Washington, DC: Trust for America's Health, 2009.

U.S. Consumer Product Safety Commission. *Carbon Monoxide Questions and Answers* (2009). Available at: http://www.cpsc.gov/CPSCPUB/PUBS/466.html. Accessed July 5, 2010.

Vilke, G.M., A.M. Smith, L.U. Ray, P.J. Steen, P.A. Murrin, and T.C. Chan. Airway obstruction in children aged less than 5 years: The prehospital experience. *Prehosp Emerg Care* 2004:8(2):196–9.

Warda, L.J., and M.F. Ballesteros. Interventions to prevent residential fire injury. In: Doll, L.S., S.E. Bonzo, J.A. Mercy, and D.A. Sleet, eds. *Handbook of Injury and Violence Prevention.* New York: Springer, 2007: pp. 97–115.

Wintemute, G.J. Childhood drowning and near-drowning in the United States. *Am J Dis Child* 1990:144(6):663–9.

Zaloshnja, E., T.R. Miller, B.A. Lawrence, and E. Romano. The costs of unintentional home injuries. *Am J Prev Med* 2005:28(1):88–94.

Reducing Health Disparity through Healthy Housing

Fatemeh Shafiei, PhD

Most Americans have benefited from improvements in health during the last century. However, not all segments of the population benefited equally, as people of color and low-income persons continue to have a disproportionate share of illnesses and face premature death and higher infant mortality rates. There are significant disparities in life expectancy and death rates between people of color and Whites (U.S. Department of Health and Human Services 2001). There are various causes for the differences in health, also known as "health disparities." According to the Centers for Disease Control and Prevention (CDC), "poverty, unequal access to health care, poor environmental conditions, educational inequalities, individual behaviors, and language barriers are all significant contributors to health disparities" (CDC 2009). According to the Surgeon General, "Many of the disparities in health status among subpopulations may be linked to poor access to safe and healthy homes, which is most prevalent among lower income populations, populations with disabilities, and minority populations" (U.S. Surgeon General 2009). The federal government has articulated its desire and commitment to achieving "health equity"; eliminating "health disparities" based on race, ethnicity, gender, and income in the nation; and improving "the health of all groups" through the second overarching goal of *Healthy People 2020*, which outlines specific objectives and sets targets to be achieved by 2020.

The social determinants of health are not a new concept in public health. At the turn of the twentieth century, scholar and civil rights activist W.E.B. DuBois documented racial disparities in health among African American and White citizens. DuBois focused on the role of social determinants, such as poor housing, sanitation, and diet (DuBois 1899). More than 100 years later, the pronounced pattern of health disparities persists. In recent decades, the emergence of better understanding of the nexus between health, environment, and poverty is revolutionizing public health. Public health professionals increasingly are realizing that addressing health disparities requires a deeper understanding of the crucial role that social determinants play—including race/ethnicity, class, and the built environment.

The link between environmental quality and health has long been recognized. According to the World Health Organization (WHO), environmental health "comprises those aspects of human health, disease, and injury that are determined or influenced by factors in the environment. This includes the study of both the direct pathological effects of various chemical, physical, and biological agents, as well as the effects on health of the broad physical and social environmental, which includes housing, urban development, land-use and transportation" (WHO 1997). The WHO reports that environmental factors contribute to approximately 23% of all global deaths and 24% of the global disease burden (Prüss-Üstün and Corvalán 2006).

This chapter uses an environmental justice prism and framework to evaluate the housing and neighborhood environments as the built/physical environmental components of social determinants of health and their role in health disparities. Healthy housing will be studied in this context. The built/physical environment can be divided into two general categories: "health-promoting environment" and "health-inhibiting environment." A health-promoting environment contains amenities/resources, access to which promote residents' health and prevents disease. A health-inhibiting environment contains environmental stressors, the exposure to which contributes to the residents' decline in health and prevalence of disease. This study demonstrates a relationship between race, ethnicity, and class on the one hand, and the likelihood of living in a "health-inhibiting environment" on the other. Asthma and lead poisoning are presented as examples, although other home hazards may be explored with this framework. This study may help formulate policies to address health disparities and design intervention strategies that target their root causes.

A preponderance of research documents that, from cradle to grave, the poor and people of color are disproportionately exposed to multiple sources of health-threatening physical environments in their homes, neighborhoods, and workplace. The right to a healthy home is considered by most Americans to be a fundamental part of the American dream. Considering the time that one generally spends in the home makes it clear that a healthy indoor environment is an important component of disease prevention. Dilapidated and substandard houses serve as contributing culprits in maintaining health disparity in the United States. "Where a person lives has tremendous social, economic, and health implications" (Bullard and Lee 1994).

Better understanding of the public health consequences of "health-promoting environments" and "health-inhibiting environments" would help us promote health and prevent housing- and neighborhood-related diseases and illnesses. "Our homes ought to be a place where we can raise our children without fear of making them sick," said U.S. Department of Housing and Urban Development (HUD) Deputy Secretary Ron Sims. "As a nation, we must think smarter about how we design, build, renovate and maintain our homes in a way that protects the health and safety of those who ultimately live in them" (HUD 2009).

ENVIRONMENTAL JUSTICE

Over the past three decades, disenfranchised populations, in their fight against environmental injustices such as siting of toxic wastes, noxious facilities, and air and water pollution, demonstrated that health is at the core of their quest for environmental justice. Environmental justice is the merging of two social movements: environmental and civil rights. Environmental justice expands the concept of civil rights by adding healthy air, water, and land to the list of rights (Bullard 1993, 2000). Environmental justice also expands the notion of environment from nature/wilderness to the built environment where people "live, work, and play" (Bullard 1993, 2000). The environmental justice movement draws a link between individual/community rights and the democratic process, and connects it to the allocation of resources. Simultaneously, the movement considers the relationship of the denial of these rights to the allocation of risks and unequal protection. Environmental justice is defined as "the principle that all people and communities are entitled to equal protection of environmental and public health laws and regulations" by Robert Bullard, director of the Environmental Justice Resource Center at Clark Atlanta University, in his now classic book *Dumping in Dixie: Race, Class, and Environmental Quality* (Bullard 2000).

The concerns articulated by the environmental justice movement served as impetus for the creation of the U.S. Environmental Protection Agency (EPA) Office of Environmental Equity, which later became the Office of Environmental Justice, and the National Environmental Justice Advisory Committee, both of which intended to serve as advising bodies to the EPA on matters of environmental justice. Environmental justice is defined by the EPA as follows: ". . . no group of people, including racial, ethnic, or socioeconomic groups should bear a disproportionate share of negative environmental consequences resulting from industrial, municipal, and commercial operations or the execution of federal, state, local, and tribal programs and policies" (U.S. EPA 1998).

A significant policy response to the concerns of the environmental justice communities was the Executive Order 12898, "Federal Actions to Address Environmental Justice in Minority Populations and Low-Income Populations," signed by President Clinton. The Executive Order directs each federal agency to "make achieving environmental justice part of its mission by identifying and addressing, as appropriate, disproportionately high and adverse human health or environmental effects of its programs, policies, and activities on minority populations and low-income populations" (Clinton 1994).

Asthma, Health Disparity, and Healthy Housing

The relationship between the prevalence, morbidity, and mortality of asthma and the inequality in race and class can be easily framed in terms of environmental justice. Asthma is in fact an environmental justice poster child. The unequal burden of the disease falls disproportionately on the shoulders of poor and minority communities. In the United States, asthma disproportionately affects minority children living in urban areas and poor children. Although the prevalence of asthma among African American children is approximately twice that of White children, emergency department visits and hospitalization rates for African American children are 3–4 times higher than those for White children. African American children are also 4–5 times more likely than White children to die of asthma. The prevalence of asthma among Hispanic children is mixed. Puerto Rican children have a higher prevalence rate of asthma than any other Hispanic subpopulations (American Lung Association 2009; Bloom, Cohen, and Freeman 2007; CDC 2009; Davis et al. 2006; Kirschstein 2000; U.S. Surgeon General 2009). Asthma thus ranks as one of the leading causes of health disparities among low-income populations and people of color.

The focus of asthma epidemiologic studies traditionally has been on family and individual risk factors. However, biological explanations for racial/ethnic disparity are insufficient because race/ethnicity is a social and not a biological construct. Scholars increasingly are focusing on the "broader social context in which individuals live" (Wright and Subramanian 2007). Scholars recommend a multilevel approach that studies asthma within the environmental, community, psycho-socioeconomic, and biological contexts. Such an approach, they argue, is likely to provide a better understanding of asthma disparities (Wright and Subramanian 2007). The new field of social epidemiology stresses the study of physical and social characteristics of neighborhood. According to this public health perspective, asthma is not determined by an "individual's biologic composition, or 'who you are,' or social context, or 'where you are,' but rather all of these factors; so, who you are depends in part on where you are" (Corburn, Osleeb, and Porter 2006).

A study of children with asthma in Boston's public housing concluded that children would benefit from public housing–based interventions aimed at reducing indoor allergens, especially cockroaches and dust mites (Levy et al. 2004). A study of inner-city minority households with young children in northern Manhattan in New York City investigated the relationship between housing deterioration and allergen levels. The study concluded that the greater the dilapidation, the higher the allergen levels. The authors recommended interventions to address social–structural aspects of housing that would reduce allergen levels (Rauh, Chew, and Garfinkel 2002). A study of urban asthma in New York City analyzed the effects of neighborhood characteristics (e.g., sociodemographics, housing conditions, and ambient air pollution) on the rate of childhood asthma hospitalization. Corburn, Osleeb, and Porter (2006) used asthma hospitalization data between 1997 and 2000 in U.S. census tracts and neighborhood characteristics, concluding that being a minority, having low-income status, and living in substandard housing were significant predictors of asthma hospitalizations. As the number of housing units that were classified as dilapidated increased, so did the rate of asthma hospitalization. In some cases there were three times more dilapidated housing units in the asthma hotspot (Corburn, Osleeb, and Porter 2006).

Controlling indoor environmental factors by providing a "health-promoting environment" can significantly affect the prevalence, morbidity, and mortality of asthma. There is no cure for asthma, so prevention is the key to reducing or eliminating its severity for those who have been diagnosed and its prevalence among those who have not. There is a preponderance of evidence showing the link between the exposure to indoor and outdoor asthma triggers and the onset and severity of asthma attacks. Studies suggest that reducing exposure to allergens (e.g., mice, cockroaches, mold, and tobacco smoke) has reduced the number of days with asthma-related symptoms and the number of school absences (Krieger et al. 2000, 2002, 2005).

Studies suggest that indoor exposure to allergens can be reduced, if not totally eliminated. It thus makes economic sense to direct efforts and resources to addressing housing problems. Intervention strategies such as healthy homes have demonstrated promising results, improving health and decreasing the economic toll of asthma. In the long run, intervention strategies that focus on housing remediation and the use of integrated pest management that reduces or eliminates exposure to indoor allergens can go a long way in reducing the disproportionate burden of asthma on poor and minority populations (National Center for Healthy Housing 2009).

Lead Poisoning, Health Disparity, and Healthy Housing

In the United States, hundreds of thousands of children are harmed by lead every year. Although fatal lead poisoning has recently almost disappeared and median blood lead concentrations have significantly decreased, lead continues to be a health problem among children in the United States (HUD 2007). Between 1999 and 2004, approximately 240,000 children 1–5 years of age had blood lead levels of 10 µg/dL or greater as the result of exposure to lead paint in and around their homes. Low-income and minority children are "more likely to be exposed to lead in their homes" (U.S. Surgeon General 2009).

Lead poisoning is a preventable disease. The familial, social, and economic toll of lead is immense. There is well-documented information about the pathways of exposure, the sources of exposure, and the ways to eliminate or reduce exposure that can prevent or reduce children's exposure to lead. There has been a clear shift to the precautionary approach of eliminating the threat *before* the harm and away from the old approach of *managing* lead poisoning. By minimizing and eliminating exposure to lead in housing, the occurrence of neurodevelopmental disability can be reduced.

Childhood lead poisoning has declined dramatically since 1976 because of laws that have banned lead use in gasoline, paint, and other products. The annual economic benefit from this dramatic reduction in lead poisoning in the United States, from increases in intelligence quotients and increased earnings resulting from workers' productivity, is estimated to be between $110 and $319 billion (Grosse et al. 2002). Despite significant progress in substantially reducing blood lead levels in U.S. children, childhood lead poisoning remains a common, yet preventable health problem (CDC 2007).

Lead poisoning is an environmental justice issue. In 2000, there were 24 million housing units with significant lead-based paint hazards, of which 1.2 million were occupied by low-income families with children younger than 6 years of age (Jacobs et al. 2002). Lead poisoning affects children across all socioeconomic levels, but because lead hazards are more prevalent in older, substandard/dilapidated housing, which is often concentrated in the inner-city neighborhoods and low-income communities of color, it disproportionately affects the poor and people of color. The risks are much higher in poorly maintained rental housing. A 2001 study of children in 2 large urban communities in Chicago with high percentages of racial/ethnic minority residents, poverty, and old housing found that the rate of lead poisoning was more than 12 times higher than the national average (Gerberding 2002).

Poor people and people of color are also at higher risk of exposure to lead not only from housing but also from ambient air emission, Superfund sites, and drinking water. The U.S. EPA under Superfund legislation is mandated to identify the nation's most dangerous hazardous waste sites, rank them according to their risk to human health and environment, and place them on the National Priority List

(NPL) for remediation. According to the Agency for Toxic Substances and Disease Registry, lead has been present in at least 1,272 of the 1,684 NPL sites (Agency for Toxic Substances and Disease Registry 2007). Children living near these sites where lead is detected are also at risk for exposure to high levels of lead (U.S. Department of Health and Human Services 2005). According to the EPA, as of September 2008, there were approximately 1.1% or 800,000 children who lived within 1 mile of NPL sites that had not been controlled or cleaned up (U.S. EPA 2003).

HEALTH-INHIBITING ENVIRONMENT: DISPARITIES IN NEIGHBORHOOD QUALITY AND DESIGN

The intersection between neighborhood environmental quality/design and health is a growing field of public health. The Surgeon General in his "Call to Action to Promote Healthy Homes" stated "[t]he surrounding neighborhood and community are also important aspects of healthy homes" (U.S. Surgeon General 2009). To shed light on the possible link between health-inhibiting environment and health disparities, this section will focus on two aspects of a neighborhood: 1) locally unwanted land uses (Bullard 2000) that contribute to the community's disproportionate exposure to pollutants and risks; and 2) lack of infrastructure and the community's deprivation of the resources/amenities. Many scholars believe that exposure to outdoor pollutants and lack of access to resources/amenities are risk factors that contribute to health disparities (Bullard 1993, 2000, 2005; Bullard and Johnson 1997; Bullard and Wright 2009; Bullard et al. 2007; Lee 1993; Wright 2003, 2005). The Agriculture Street Landfill in New Orleans, where homes and school were built on landfills, exemplifies the disproportionate exposure to pollutants and risks. Although the case of Agricultural Street Landfill is compelling, the snapshot of studies documenting that low-income communities and communities of color are disproportionately exposed to pollutants reveals that the case is not an anomaly.

The Agriculture Street Landfill

New Orleans' Agricultural Street community, the two mostly African American Gordon Plaza and Press Park subdivisions, was built on the portion of the land that was a municipal landfill for decades. New Orleans dumped its garbage from 1910 to 1966 into Agricultural Street Landfill, approximately 190 acres in the Ninth Ward. The site was also used for dumping the debris from Hurricane Betsy, which struck New Orleans in 1965. Press Park, consisting of 167 public housing units, was part of the federal government's home ownership program designed to assist lower-income families to purchase homes. In 1977, HUD and the Housing

Authority of New Orleans expanded the plan, and the construction for Gordon Plaza, the second subdivision consisting of 67 single-family homes, started. In 1986, the U.S. EPA conducted a site inspection of the Agriculture Street Landfill neighborhood and found lead, zinc, mercury, cadmium, and arsenic. However, according to the Hazard Ranking System (HRS) in use at the EPA at that time, the score was not high enough to trigger any regulatory action. In 1990, in response to the passage of the Superfund Amendment and Reauthorization Act of 1986, the EPA revised its HRS model (Bullard and Wright 2009; Wright and Bullard 2007; Leiker 2001). In 1993, the EPA performed an Expanded Site Inspection, and in 1994 the Agriculture Street Landfill, on the basis of its HRS rank according to its risk to human health and environment, was identified as one of the nation's dangerous hazardous waste sites and placed on the NPL for remediation. Despite residents' demand for property buy-out and relocation, the EPA opted for the $20 million clean-up of the site and completed it in 2001.

In 1983, part of the Agricultural Street Landfill was acquired by the Orleans Parish School Board. Despite concerns over the contamination and presence of heavy metals on the site, the construction plan for building a school moved forward. In 1989, Moton Elementary public school, built at a cost of $8 million, opened with 421 students (Bullard and Wright 2009; Wright and Bullard 2007; Leiker 2001). Residents unhappy with the EPA's clean-up decision filed a class-action lawsuit against the city of New Orleans, its housing authority, and its school board for relocation and damages (Bullard and Wright 2009).

Approximately one year after Hurricane Katrina, the city of New Orleans received a "clean bill of health" with one exception—the Agricultural Street Landfill neighborhood (Bullard and Wright 2009). Despite the cleanup of the site in 2001, the EPA found dangerous levels of cancer-causing chemicals in residents' yards. Residents were supplied Federal Emergency Management Agency (FEMA) travel trailers. Not long after, there were reports that FEMA-supplied trailers used by displaced Katrina residents were toxic and releasing potentially dangerous levels of formaldehyde, a carcinogen. In August of 2007, FEMA started moving families out of the trailers and into rental housing (Bullard and Wright 2009). In 2006, Civil District Court Judge Nadine Ramsey ruled in favor of residents, declaring the neighborhood "unreasonably dangerous" and "uninhabitable." The ruling was upheld by the Louisiana Supreme Court in July of 2008 (Bullard and Wright 2009).

Unequal Exposure to Pollutants

The Mississippi River chemical corridor, where 135 petrochemical plants operate in the 85-mile stretch between Baton Rouge and New Orleans in Louisiana, also known as "Cancer Alley," exemplifies the effects of living in proximity to pollutants. The air, land, and water along the corridor contained so many carcino-gens that at one point the area was characterized as a "massive human experi-ment" (Wright 2003, 2005). This section provides snapshots of selected reports and studies documenting that people of color and those living in poverty are dispro-portionately exposed to pollution. Reports of the disproportionate burden of envi-ronmental hazards on the poor and communities of color started mounting in the 1970s. As early as 1971, the President's Council on Environmental Quality annual report acknowledged that racial discrimination had adverse impacts on urban poor and the quality of their environment. In 1979, an African American community in Houston, Texas, filed the *Bean v. Southwestern Waste Management, Inc.*, lawsuit, the first civil rights suit challenging the siting of a solid waste facility (Bullard 2000). But it was not until 1982, when the predominantly African American com-munity in Warren County, North Carolina, protested the siting of a polychlorinated biphenyl landfill in their community, that environmental justice began to capture national attention and serve as an impetus for mobilization against environmental injustices (Bullard 2000). Five years later, the United Church of Christ (UCC) Com-mission for Racial Justice's 1987 landmark study *Toxic Wastes and Race in the United States* concluded that race was the most important factor in the location of the toxic waste sites (UCC 1987). The study showed that Warren County was far from being an isolated incident.

The UCC's study was revisited in 2007, its twentieth anniversary. A 2007 update to this work, *Toxic Wastes and Race at Twenty 1987–2007*, further con-firmed the findings of the earlier UCC study. The study used distance-based meth-ods, current databases for commercial hazardous facilities, and data from the 2000 Census to assess the correlation between the racial and socioeconomic makeup of the community and the siting of the facilities. Among other findings, the study noted that people of color constituted the majority (56%) of the people living in neighborhoods within 1.8 miles of hazardous waste facilities and that neighbor-hoods of color were more likely (69%) to have clustered facilities. The study con-cluded that environmental injustice was more prevalent than two decades earlier; racial and socioeconomic disparities in the location of hazardous waste facilities were widespread; neighborhoods and communities of color had greater concentra-tions of commercial hazardous sites than found in the 1987 study; and race was the most significant predictor of the location of these facilities (Bullard et al. 2007).

"More than sixty-eight percent of African Americans live within 30 miles of a coal-fired power plant—the distance within which the maximum effects of the smokestack plume are expected to occur." This is compared with "fifty-six percent of white Americans" (Clear the Air et al. 2002). Coal-fired power plants are among the largest industrial sources of air pollution in the United States. They emit vast amounts of ozone, particulate matter, sulfur dioxide, and nitrogen oxides, which are respiratory irritants and contribute to respiratory problems, including asthma.

An *Associated Press* analysis (Pace 2005) concluded that African Americans are "79 percent more likely than whites to live in neighborhoods where industrial pollution is suspected of posing the greatest health danger." The study concluded that "Residents in neighborhoods with the highest pollution scores also tend to be poorer, less educated and more often unemployed than those elsewhere in the country." According to Carol Browner, the U.S. EPA's former administrator, "Poor communities, frequently communities of color but not exclusively, suffer disproportionately" (Pace 2005).

Health-Inhibiting Environment: Neighborhood Infrastructure and Unequal Access/Scarcity of Resources

Although there is an abundance of toxic-waste sites and air pollution in communities comprising low-income people and people of color, there is a serious scarcity of amenities and resources in those communities. Environmental justice is expanding to include not only the hazards that exist in the communities of color but also the lack of amenities, such as healthy food. There is no shortage of liquor stores, fast-food operations, and store-front grocery stores in the inner-city neighborhoods. Gottlieb, an environmental justice and urban planning scholar, suggests that the expansion of the environmental justice agenda should include "food justice." He urges that the environmental justice slogan of "where we live, work, and play" be expanded to include "where, what, and how we eat." He argues that food justice is associated with communities' health and access to healthy foods such as fresh fruit and vegetables, which can help prevent diet-related diseases. Furthermore, he states that "food deserts" in low-income communities have contributed to a lack of access to fresh, affordable, and healthy food with "direct health and nutritional consequences" (Gottlieb 2009).

Lack of access to green space, parks, and neighborhood outdoor spaces has significant health implications. Children living in inner-city neighborhoods are more dependent on parks and open/green spaces than the children of suburban residents. At the same time, social and environmental risks significantly compromise the ability of low-income and inner-city residents to use neighborhood parks and playgrounds. The "cumulative disadvantageous risks" of "crime, drugs, gang activities, systemic poverty, traffic dangers, and pollution" have been found to produce "social-psychological factors that may influence children's current and future behavior" (Outley 2006).

Studies associate access to parks and open space to public health. During 2003–2004, the prevalence of obesity among African American females aged 2–19 years was 24% compared with 15% for White females (CDC 2009). Scholars assert that one of the contributing factors to obesity in children in the communities of color in Los Angeles, California, is the unavailability of parks (Garcia and Flores 2005).

There are significant disparities in terms of access to insurance for the poor and people of color. According to the Census Bureau, there are more than 45 million people who are without health insurance, including more than 8 million children. Poor children are more likely to be uninsured. In 2007, the uninsured rate was higher for minority children than for White children. The rates of uninsured were 7.3% for White children, 20.0% for Hispanic children, 12.2% for African American children, and 11.7% for Asian children. The uninsured rates were also higher for minority adults than for White adults. The rates of uninsured were 10.4% for White adults, 32.1% for Hispanic adults, and 19.5% for African American adults (U.S. Census Bureau 2008).

PRECAUTIONARY PRINCIPLE AND HEALTHY HOUSING

The Constitution of the WHO defines health as "a state of complete physical, mental, and social well-being, not just merely an absence of disease or infirmity" (WHO 2007). For too long, the dominant health care paradigm in the United States has been treating disease and finding cures with most of the national expenditure on health care going to providing medical care and biomedical research. This reactive policy of waiting until harm was done has been costly, with unintended consequences. In a report by Trust for America's Health, the researchers concluded that for every dollar invested in prevention, the country will save $5.60. If the nation invested $10 per person in prevention, it would save the nation $18 billion in 5 years (Trust for America's Health 2008). This rate of return for investment in prevention is remarkable. In North Carolina alone, the 1-year price tag of substandard housing–related diseases, disabilities, and injuries among children is approximately $95 million (HUD 2008).

There is a growing recognition that housing-related hazards, such as lead, pesticides, carbon monoxide, safety hazards, radon, mold, and allergens, greatly affect residents' health. However, as asthma and lead poisoning demonstrate, the public health policy of managing and regulating risks does not work. As Albert Einstein once remarked, "We can't solve problems by using the same kind of thinking we used when we created them." We stand at the brink of a new era of a public health paradigm of disease prevention. Healthy housing adds significant momentum to this health paradigm of disease prevention and helps the nation to make serious strides toward reducing and alleviating health disparity.

"When an activity raises threats of harm to human health or the environment, precautionary measures should be taken even if some cause and effect relationships are not fully established scientifically" (Schettler, Barrett, and Raffensperger 2002). The Precautionary Principle proposes a proactive policy of precautionary action: taking preventive measures to protect public health and putting in place proactive policies instead of corrective and reactive policies. The Surgeon General defines a "healthy home" as one that is "sited, designed, built, renovated, and maintained in ways that support the health of residents" (U.S. Surgeon General 2009). Achieving what is necessary for healthy people requires thinking out of the box, moving beyond compartmentalization of the problems, and moving toward system thinking, integrating, connecting, and finding synergies between public health and environmental and social policies. In this sense, one can conclude that healthy housing is a forward-looking, proactive policy that would create this synergy. Healthy housing moves away from risk management and shifts into prevention that is compatible with the Precautionary Principle and the environmental justice framework that "adopts a public health model of prevention (elimination of the threat before harm occurs) as the preferred strategy" (Bullard 2000).

BARRIERS TO MAKING HEALTHY HOUSING AFFORDABLE AND ACCESSIBLE

On June 9, 2009, healthy housing gained significant momentum with the Surgeon General's "Call to Action to Promote Healthy Homes." HUD started the Healthy Homes Initiative more than a decade earlier. However, healthy homes remain elusive for the majority of the poor and people of color. Achieving environmental justice goals as expressed in Executive Order 12898 needs to be specifically articulated and incorporated with designated milestones in healthy homes policy. However, achieving the goals and objectives of healthy homes requires meaningful appropriations and allocation of resources. The biggest challenge for policy makers and federal and state governments is to make healthy homes accessible and affordable. To this end, significant resources and institutional changes are needed.

There are significant challenges in obtaining an adequate supply of affordable healthy homes and making them available to people who need them. In 2007, there were 37.5 million people living in poverty, 13.3 million of whom were children. The poverty rate was much higher for minority people. The rates were 8.2% for Whites, 24.5% for African Americans, 21.5% for Hispanics, and 10.2% for Asians (U.S. Census Bureau 2008). Poverty poses a significant challenge for achieving healthy housing because necessary maintenance gets deferred.

According to the 2007 American Housing Survey, there are more than 5.7 million homes with severe or moderate physical problems (U.S. Census Bureau 2008). Poor people confronted with a choice between housing affordability and health often chose affordability.

There is a significant shortage of affordable housing. Eighteen million families spend more than 50% of their income on housing. This reflects a surge of approximately 4 million from 2001 to 2006. This surge was the outcome of the increase in housing costs without real income growth. As a result, other essential expenses suffered, such as food, clothing, and medical care (Joint Center for Housing Studies of Harvard University 2008).

There are an estimated 4.4 million homeless people in the United States; among them 1.3 million are children (U.S. Surgeon General 2009). Numerous studies demonstrate that affordable housing is crucial in ending homelessness. Research has shown that 80% of homeless families that received "housing subsidy or public housing remained stably housed" (National Alliance to End Homelessness 2007). Studies also support the belief that the benefits of affordable housing are shared by the community at large. Research examining the relationship between "quality affordable housing" and benefit to the larger community has found that "quality affordable housing" is associated with better health and better educational performance. This is contrary to the opponents' claim that affordable housing and mixed development threaten neighborhood property values and contain no benefit for the community (Mueller and Tighe 2007).

CONCLUSION

This chapter discussed the link between racial/ethnic/class disparities and the propensity of living in health-inhibiting environments. Very often the challenge is to find reliable and valid data correlating environmental risk factors to adverse health outcomes. However, in this case, numerous cited studies provided a strong link between exposure and the prevalence of disease. The cited studies confirm that the differential exposure to allergens and pollutants present in substandard/dilapidated housing contributes to the prevalence of asthma and lead poisoning among minority and poor populations. Understanding this link can help us better design targeted intervention strategies, among them healthy homes, to reduce or avert the public health problems that contribute to health disparities.

The current piecemeal approach of directing resources to address a single health problem, such as asthma or lead poisoning, is inefficient, expensive, and inadequate. Healthy housing advances system thinking in addressing health issues. Adopting public health policies that limit, and better yet prevent, exposure to harmful substances is an essential course of action. Although no single strategy can completely solve the complex and multilayered causes of health disparities in the nation, improving housing and neighborhood conditions is a major step in the right direction.

REFERENCES

Agency for Toxic Substances and Disease Registry. *Lead*. Atlanta, GA: Agency for Toxic Substances and Disease Registry, 2007. Case #7439-92-1.

American Lung Association, Epidemiology and Statistics Unit, Research and Program Services. *Trends in Asthma Morbidity and Mortality*. 2009. Available at: http://www.lungusa.org/finding-cures/our-research/trend-reports/asthma-trend-report.pdf. Accessed July 30, 2010.

Bloom, B., R.A. Cohen, and G. Freeman. *Summary Health Statistic for U.S. Children: National Health Interview Survey, 2007*. Atlanta, GA: U.S. Department of Health and Human Services, CDC, NCHS, 2009 (Series 10, Number 239). Available at: http://www.cdc.gov/nchs/data/series/sr_10/sr10_239.pdf. Accessed June 30, 2009.

Bullard, R.D., ed. *Confronting Environmental Racism: Voices from the Grassroots*. Boston, MA: South End Press, 1993.

——. *Dumping in Dixie: Race, Class, and Environmental Quality*. 3rd ed. Boulder, CO: Westview Press, 2000:xiv, 123.

——. Environmental justice in the twenty-first century. In: Bullard, R.D., ed. *The Quest for Environmental Justice: Human Rights and the Politics of Pollution*. San Francisco, CA: Sierra Club Books, 2005:26.

Bullard, R.D., and G.S. Johnson, eds. *Just Transportation: Dismantling Race and Class Barriers to Mobility*. Montpelier, VT: New Society Publishers, 1997.

Bullard, R.D., and B. Wright. Race, place, and the environment in the post-Katrina New Orleans. In: Bullard, R.D., and B. Wright, eds. *Race, Place, and Environmental Justice after Hurricane Katrina: Struggle to Reclaim, Rebuild, and Revitalize New Orleans and the Gulf Coast*. Boulder, CO: Westview Press, 2009:19–47.

Bullard, R. D., and C. Lee. Introduction: Racism and American Apartheid. In: Bullard, R. D., J. E. Grigsby III, and C. Lee, eds. *Residential Apartheid: The American Legacy*. Los Angeles, CA: UCLA Center for Afro-American Studies, 1994:7.

Bullard, R.D., P. Mohai, R. Saha, and B. Wright. *Toxic Wastes and Race at Twenty 1987–2007*. Cleveland, OH: United Church of Christ, 2007. This report was prepared for the United Church of Christ Justice and Witness Ministries. Available at: http://www.ejrc.cau.edu/TWART%20Final.pdf. Accessed March 20, 2009.

Centers for Disease Control and Prevention (CDC) Advisory Committee on Childhood Lead Poisoning Prevention. Interpreting and managing blood lead levels < 10μg/dl in children and reducing childhood exposures to lead: Recommendations of CDC's Advisory Committee on Childhood Lead Poisoning Prevention. *MMWR Recomm Rep* (2007):56:(RR-8):1–16. Available at: http://www.cdc.gov/mmwr/preview/mmwrhtml/rr5608a1.htm#tab1. Accessed June 23, 2009.

Centers for Disease Control and Prevention. *Health Disparities and Racial/Ethnic Minority Youth* (2009). Available at: http://www.cdc.gov/Features/HealthDisparities. Accessed July 15, 2010.

Clear the Air, the Black Leadership Forum (BLF), the Southern Organizing Committee for Economic and Social Justice (SOC), and the Georgia Coalition for the Peoples' Agenda (GCPA). *Air of Injustice: African Americans and Power Plant Pollution.* Orlando, FL: LaBerge Printers, Inc., 2002. Available at: http://www.catf.us/publications/reports/AirofInjustice.pdf. Accessed May 9, 2009.

Clinton, W.J. Executive Order 12898. Federal Actions to Address Environmental Justice in Minority Populations and Low-Income Populations. Reg 59:7629, 1994:1. Available at: http://www.epa.gov/Region2/ej/exec_order_12898.pdf. Accessed June 8, 2009.

Corburn, J., J. Osleeb, and M. Porter. Urban asthma and the neighbourhood environment in New York City. *Health Place* (2006):12(2)167–79. Epub 2005 Jan 21.

Davis, A., R. Kreutzer, M. Lipsett, G. King, N. Shaikh. Asthma prevalence in Hispanic and Asian American ethnic subgroups: Results from the California Healthy Kids Survey. *Pediatrics* (2006):118(2):e363–70.

DuBois, W.E.B. *The Philadelphia Negro.* Philadelphia: Published for the University. 1899:148. Available at: http://pds.lib.harvard.edu/pds/view/2574418?n=22&s=6. Accessed March 10, 2009.

Garcia, R., and E.A. Flores. Anatomy of the urban parks movement: Equal justice, democracy, and livability in Los Angeles. In: Bullard, R.D., ed. *The Quest for Environmental Justice: Human Rights and the Politics of Pollution.* San Francisco, CA: Sierra Club Books, 2005:145–67.

Gerberding, J.L. *CDC Report to Congress for Fiscal Years 2001-2002: Childhood Lead Poisoning Prevention Activities Under Lead Contamination Control Act of 1988* (2002). Available at: http://www.cdc.gov/nceh/lead/Legislation%20&%20Policy/Reporttocongress(2001-2002).pdf. Accessed July 6, 2009.

Gottlieb, R. Where we live, work, play . . . and eat: Expanding the environmental justice agenda. *Environmental Justice* (2009):2(1):7–8.

Grosse, S.D., T.D. Matte, J. Schwartz, and R.J. Jackson. Economic gains resulting from the reduction in children's exposure to lead in the U.S. *Environ Health Perspect*

(2002):110:(6):563–9. Available at: http://www.ehponline.org/members/2002/110p563-569-grosse/EHP110p563PDF.PDF. Accessed April 10, 2009.

Jacobs, D.E., R. P. Clickner, J.Y. Zhou, et al. The prevalence of lead-based paint hazards in U.S. housing. *Environ Health Perspect* (2002):110(10):A599–606.

Joint Center for Housing Studies of Harvard University. *The State of the Nation's Housing 2008*. Cambridge, MA: President and Fellows of Harvard College, 2008. Available at: http://www.jchs.harvard.edu/publications/markets/son2008/son2008.pdf. Accessed June 10, 2009.

Kirschstein, R.L., National Institutes of Health, U.S. Department of Health and Human Services. *Testimony on Health Disparities: Bridging the Gap*. Before the Senate Subcommittee on Public Health, Committee on Health, Education, Labor and Pensions (July 26, 2000). Available at: http://www.hhs.gov/asl/testify/t000726b.html. Accessed June 23, 2009.

Krieger, J.W., L. Song, T.K. Takaro, and J. Stout, Asthma and the home environment of low-income urban children: Preliminary findings from the Seattle-King County healthy homes project. *J Urban Health* (2000):77(1):50–67.

Krieger, J.W, T.K. Takaro, C. Allen, L. Song, and M. Weaver. The Seattle-King County Healthy Homes Project: A randomized, controlled trial of community health worker intervention to decrease exposure to indoor asthma triggers. *Am J Public Health* (2005):95(4):652–9.

Krieger, J., T.K. Takaro, C. Allen, et al. The Seattle-King County Healthy Homes Project: Implementation of a comprehensive approach to improving indoor environmental quality for low-income children with asthma. *Environ Health Perspect* (2002):110(Suppl 2):311–22.

Lee, C. Beyond toxic wastes and race. In: Bullard, R.D., ed. *Confronting Environmental Racism: Voices from the Grassroots*, Boston, MA: South End Press, 1993:41–52.

Leiker, A. Stress and the politics of living on a Superfund site: The agricultural street municipal landfill getting the lead out of the community. In: Roberts, J.T, and M. M. Toffolon-Weiss, eds. *Chronicles from the Environmental Justice Frontline*. Cambridge, UK: Cambridge University Press, 2001:165–88.

Levy, J.I., L.K. Welker-Hood, J.E. Clougherty, R.E. Dodson, S. Steinbach, and H.P. Hynes. Lung function, asthma symptoms, and quality of life for children in public housing in Boston: A case series analysis. *Environ Health* 2004:3(1):13. Available at: http://www.ehjournal.net/content/pdf/1476-069X-3-13.pdf. Accessed June 29, 2009.

Mueller, E.J., and J.R. Tighe. Making the case for affordable housing: Connecting housing with health and education outcome. *J Plann Lit* (2007):21(4):371–85.

National Alliance to End Homelessness. *Policy Guide* (July 2007). Available at: http://crossroadsri.org/pdf/NAEH-2007_Homeless_Policy_Guide.pdf. Accessed March 15, 2009.

National Center for Healthy Housing. *Housing Interventions and Health Outcomes: A Review of the Evidence* (2009). Available at: http://www.nchh.org/Research/Archived-Research-Projects/Housing-Interventions-and-Health-Outcomes.aspx. Accessed March 9, 2010.

Outley, C.W. The challenges of environmental risks for children: The impact of cumulative disadvantageous risks. *George Wright Forum* (2006):23(4):49–56.

Pace, D. AP: More blacks live with pollution. *The Associated Press*, December 13, 2005. Available at: http://hosted.ap.org/specials/interactives/archive/pollution/part1.html. Accessed on July 12, 2009.

Prüss-Üstün, A., and C. Corvalán. *Preventing Disease through Healthy Environments: Toward an Estimate of the Environmental Burden of Disease*. Geneva, Switzerland: WHO, 2006:9.

Rauh, V.A., G.R. Chew, and R.S. Garfinkel. Deteriorated housing contributes to high cockroach allergen levels in inner-city households. *Environ Health Perspect* (2002):110(Suppl 2):323–7.

Schettler, T., K. Barrett, and C. Raffensperger. The precautionary principle: A guide for protecting public health and the environment. In: McCally, M., ed. *Life Support: The Environment and Human Health*. Cambridge, MA: The MIT Press, 2002:241.

Trust for America's Health. *Prevention for a Healthier America: Investments in Disease Prevention Yield Significant Savings, Stronger Communities* (July 2008). Available at: http://healthyamericans.org/reports/prevention08/Prevention08.pdf. Accessed July 12, 2009.

The United Church of Christ Commission for Racial Justice. *Toxic Wastes and Race in the United States: A National Report on the Racial and Socioeconomic Characteristics of Communities with Hazardous Waste Sites*. New York: United Church of Christ, 1987.

U.S. Census Bureau. *Income, Poverty, and Health Insurance Coverage in the United States: 2007*. Washington, DC: Government Printing Office, 2008. Available at: http://www.census.gov/prod/2008pubs/p60-235.pdf. Accessed July 11, 2009.

U.S. Department of Health and Human Services. Agency for Toxic Substances and Disease Registry. *Toxicological Profile for Lead: Draft for Public Comment*. Washington, DC: Government Printing Office, 2005:349.

——. *Closing the Health Gap: Reducing Health Disparities Affecting African-Americans* (2001.11.19a). Fact Sheet. Available at: http://www.hhs.gov/news/press/2001pres/20011119a.html. Accessed July 11, 2009.

U.S. Department of Housing and Urban Development. *News Release: HUD and Acting Surgeon General Unveil National Strategy to Produce Healthy Homes* (June 9, 2009:1). Available at: http://www.hud.gov/news/release.cfm?content=pr09-083.cfm. Accessed June 10, 2009.

——. Office of Healthy Homes and Lead Hazard Control. Lead Brochure (2007). Available at: http://www.hud.gov/offices/lead/library/hhi/Lead.pdf. Accessed July 15, 2010.

——. Office of Policy Development and Research. Healthier homes, healthier children. *Research Works* 2008:5(9): 2 . Available at: http://www.huduser.org/periodicals/research works/ResearchWorks_oct_08.pdf. Accessed July 6, 2009.

U.S. Environmental Protection Agency. *Guidance for Incorporating Environmental Justice in EPA's NEPA Compliance Analysis*. Washington, DC: Government Printing Office, 1998:7. Available at: http://www.epa.gov/compliance/resources/policies/ej/ej_guidance_nepa_epa0498.pdf. Accessed June 10, 2009.

———. Measure E9: Hazardous Waste Sites (updated July 2, 2009). *America's Children and the Environment (ACE)* (2003). Available at: http://www.epa.gov/economics/children/contaminants/e9-graph.htm. Accessed July 30, 2009.

U.S. Surgeon General. *Call to Action to Promote Healthy Homes*. Washington, DC: U.S. Department of Health and Human Services, 2009:15; 13; vii. Available at: http://www.surgeongeneral.gov/topics/healthyhomes/calltoactiontopromotehealthyhomes.pdf. Accessed July 12, 2009.

World Health Organization (WHO). *Health of Indigenous Peoples* (2007). Fact Sheet No. 326. Available at: http://www.who.int/mediacentre/factsheets/fs326/en/print.html. Accessed July 28, 2009.

———. *Indicators for Policy and Decision Making in Environmental Health* (Draft). Geneva, Switzerland: WHO, 1997. In: U.S. Department of Health and Human Services. *Healthy People 2010: Understanding and Improving Health. Focus Area 8: Environmental Health*. Washington, DC: Government Printing Office, 2000:3. Available at: http://www.healthypeople.gov/Document/pdf/Volume1/08Environmental.pdf. Accessed May 10, 2009.

Wright, B. Living and dying in Louisiana's "Cancer Alley." In: Bullard, R.D., ed. *The Quest for Environmental Justice: Human Rights and the Politics of Pollution*. San Francisco, CA: Sierra Club Books, 2005:87–107.

———. Race, politics and pollution: Environmental justice in the Mississippi River chemical corridor. In: Agyeman, J., R.D. Bullard, and B. Evan, eds. *Just Sustainabilities: Development in the Unequal World*. Cambridge, MA: The MIT Press, 2003:125–45.

Wright, B., and R.D. Bullard. Wrong complexion for protection: Will the "mother of all toxic cleanups" in post-Katrina New Orleans be fair? In: Bullard, R.D., P. Mohai, R. Saha, and B. Wright, eds. *Toxic Wastes and Race at Twenty 1987–2007*. Cleveland, OH: United Church of Christ, 2007:116–25. Available at: http://www.ejrc.cau.edu/TWART%20Final.pdf. Accessed March 20, 2009.

Wright, R.J., and S.V. Subramanian. Advancing a multilevel framework for epidemiologic research on asthma disparities. *Chest* (2007):132(5 Suppl):757S–69.

Healthy Homes: The Role of Health Care Professionals

Jerome Paulson, MD, FAAP, and
Megan Sandel, MD, MPH, FAAP

Making house calls is no longer a part of practice for the majority of health care professionals in the United States (Kao et al. 2009). However, understanding the environment in which people live—in a box under the bridge, a tent in an encampment, a car, a trailer, a single-family dwelling, a multi-family dwelling—can contribute to delivering better health care services. This chapter will focus on aspects of the home environment that influence physical health of the occupants: humidity, water intrusion, chemicals, temperature, molds, indoor air pollution, or the presence of metals. We will look at various outcomes, including allergies, asthma, cancer, adverse developmental outcomes, and other issues. We will provide guidance to the practitioner on how to capture relevant information in the history and physical examination of the patient and how to use community resources to collect information about the specific home. Individuals who are poor or in racial or ethnic minority groups are more likely to experience environmental exposures in general and to live in poor housing. It is important to take these factors into account when evaluating environmental exposures and advocating at the individual and social levels (Fullilove 2001; Gee and Payne-Sturges 2004; Hood 2005; Payne-Sturges and Gee 2006; Payne-Sturges et al. 2006; see Chapter 4).

PATIENT EVALUATION

The age and developmental or cognitive status of the patient matters. Environmental factors in the home can affect the health of all individuals irrespective of their age, health status, or developmental or cognitive status. However, the age, gender, genotype, preexisting health status, and developmental or cognitive status of an individual—from preconception to death—influence how the environment affects that individual's health, the outcomes of that interaction, and how the individual interacts with the environment. There are specific populations that may be at greater risk, such as the child in utero, children, elderly individuals, and individuals with preexisting health conditions. One example of differences in vulnerability is exposure to carbon monoxide (CO), which can be more deadly for infants because they breathe in CO faster per body mass, whereas the ill effects of CO can be felt longer in the elderly, who excrete carboxyhemoglobin slower than other adults. The differences that influence children's exposures and their responses to those exposures have been extensively reviewed (Etzel and Balk 2006).

Critical Windows of Vulnerability

Timing of exposure influences outcome. In embryonic or fetal stages, some narrow "critical windows of exposure"—highly susceptible periods of organogenesis—have been defined. Although one might expect that there are other "critical windows," none are known, and this area is the subject of intense investigation (Weiss and Landrigan 2000).

PRENATAL EXPOSURES MATTER

The consideration of environmental influences that have an impact on an individual must begin before the birth of the mother of that individual. Exposure of a female fetus to environmental toxicants can influence her ova, which in turn can influence the outcome of her offspring a generation later. One example is diethylstilbestrol, from which there have been descriptions of second-generational effects in animals and humans (Blatt et al. 2003; Brouwers et al. 2006; Newbold et al. 1998, 2000). Male exposures to a number of chemicals, particularly various pesticides, have been associated with abnormalities in sperm quality and quantity, spontaneous abortions in the wives of exposed workers, and altered sex ratio in offspring (Woodruff et al. 2008). There is also evidence that male exposure to dioxins or pesticides contaminated with dioxins can lead to neural tube defects in offspring (Hansen 2008). Materials stored in the mother's body from earlier in her life (e.g., lead) and materials that she is exposed to during pregnancy (e.g., lead, pesticides, nicotine, methylmercury, and other substances) are associated with and can cause adverse pregnancy outcomes or adverse outcomes in children (Selevan, Kimmel, and Mendola 2000; Wigle et al. 2007).

KIDS ARE DIFFERENT

Children are not little adults. When children are born, some organs are not fully formed and mature at different rates over time, for example, the tonsils and other components of the reticuloendothelial system reach adult size between the ages 4 and 6 years, whereas the pulmonary tree continues to arborize and develop additional alveoli until the late teen years. Brains do not fully develop until the age of 25 years.

The surface area-to-body mass ratio is greater in children; therefore, topical exposures can result in a higher dose per unit of body weight than in an adult. In children less than 1 year of age, this is compounded by the fact that their skin permeability is greater than that of an older child or an adult.

Children, particularly in their early years, eat differently, drink differently, and breathe differently than adults. Breast milk— although the best source of nutrition for infants—may be contaminated with pesticides, lead, persistent organic pollutants, and other substances (Thundiyil, Solomon, and Miller 2007). Children eat more food and drink more water per unit of body weight than do adults (National Academy of Sciences 1993). The respiratory minute ventilation—inspired air per unit time adjusting for weight—is greater in young children than in adults (Makri et al. 2004). The implication is that when eating contaminated food, drinking contaminated water, or breathing contaminated air, children will get a higher dose per unit body weight than an adult.

There are changes in the neurologic, gastrointestinal, renal, hepatic, and endocrine systems. In the brain, both in utero and after birth, multiple processes that are susceptible to interruption by environmental toxicants occur: cellular migration, synaptogenesis, myelination, and apoptosis. There is a limited ability to repair or regenerate components of the central nervous system, and the blood–brain barrier becomes less permeable to xenobiotics over time (Hansen 2008). A child less than 2 years of age absorbs and retains a greater proportion of the amount of lead ingested orally than an older child and an adult (Ziegler et al. 1978). The cytochrome P450, one of the major detoxifying mechanisms, is inducible in adults but not in children. Glomerular filtration and tubular secretion are lower in infants, reaching adult levels at approximately 1 year of age. The endocrine system undergoes major changes during puberty, making it very different in childhood than adulthood. The time of the change may be a particular period of vulnerability.

Children's behavior changes with age (Moya, Bearer, and Etzel 2004). Infants are incapable of independent locomotion, making it impossible to remove themselves from environmental hazards such as heat and cold. Children of all ages spend more time on the floor or ground than adults. Therefore, children will come into more contact with toxins that are on or near the floor, such as lead dust or pesticides sprayed on the floor. Adolescents become more like adults and often go to work or work at home, leading to environmental exposures that one might not normally expect in "children." In a home environment, this "workplace exposure" may include household cleaning supplies.

ELDERLY INDIVIDUALS ARE DIFFERENT

Many elderly people have a dangerous confluence of housing hazards, chronic medical conditions, and loss of function. People aged more than 65 years are more likely to live in older homes that have deferred maintenance and lack safety modifications (Golant 2008; Joint Center for Housing Studies of Harvard University 2003; Newman 2003). Elderly individuals spend larger amounts of time at home as they lose mobility and have decreased social interactions as a result of aging, disability, and death of peers. Decreased mobility can contribute to more falls (Stevens, Mack, Paulozzi, and Ballesteros 2008). Also, elders are at higher risk of death at home, whether from exacerbations of respiratory illnesses (U.S. Department of Health and Human Services 2009) or extremes of heat and cold stress (Centers for Disease Control [CDC] 1988). Elders have differing sensitivities to air pollution according to their age, lung function, and underlying disease (Viegi et al. 2004). The expected rapid increase in the number of elderly in the United States in the coming decades is likely to magnify these problems (Federal Interagency Forum on Aging-Related Statistics 2006). Children and the elderly are likely to spend significant amounts of time in the same home environments because of provision of child care; co-residence; and foster, adoptive, and kinship care (Hughes et al. 2007).

MEDICAL HISTORY

In taking a medical history from a patient with a suspected dwelling-related health problem, one should complete the same history, family history, social history, developmental history (or mental status history, depending on age), work history, and review of systems as for any other patient. Children may be legally employed, in some instances as young as 11 years of age, and children living on farms may work on the farm at even younger ages (Pollack 2001). Also, one should gather information about potential environmental exposures at home, in the neighborhood, and at homes or facilities where the patient may spend appreciable amounts of time, such as relatives' homes, child care centers, schools, or adult day care centers. One also should obtain an environmental history of those buildings and information about industries in the neighborhood.

For pediatric patients, several resources exist to guide information collection (Agency for Toxic Substances and Disease Registry 2008a and 2008b; American Academy of Pediatrics Committee on Environmental Health 2006; Goldman,

Shannon, and Woolf 1999). The National Center for Healthy Housing provides online training specifically for the Pediatric Environmental Home Assessment (http://www.healthyhomestraining.org/Nurse/PEHA_Start.htm) (Table 5.1).

The Agency for Toxic Substances and Disease Registry has an extensive online training program focused on taking an environmental health history from individuals of all ages (Agency for Toxic Substances and Disease Registry Case Studies 2008a). A long and detailed Exposure History Form from that document is reproduced in Table 5.2. For the primary care practitioner, adopting components of this document may be the most expedient way of using it.

There are several important questions that should be raised as one takes a history, each of which has an associated housing hazard:

- What are the age and condition of the home? Is there lead, mold, or asbestos?
- Is there an ongoing or planned renovation?
- Are CO detectors and smoke alarms installed?
- What type of heating/air conditioning system does the home have?
- Where and how are chemicals and pesticides stored?
- Has the home been tested for radon?

WHAT ARE THE AGE AND CONDITION OF THE HOME? IS THERE LEAD, MOLD, OR ASBESTOS?

Lead

Lead paint was used in home construction until the late 1970s. Buildings constructed before 1950 are most likely to have leaded paint that may peel, chip, or chalk. Lead dust can be released from poorly maintained surfaces and windows and doors because of the friction of opening and closing.

Mold

It is not water but the water damage to buildings and building materials that is related to health problems. Excess water from a broken pipe or leaky roof, or improperly drained condensate from an air conditioner, can damage building materials such as wallboard, underlayments, and carpet. Although the chief complaint about a building is often the growth of mold, water-damaged materials in and of themselves may release hazardous substances and the water contributes to the growth of bacteria as well as mold.

The primary health hazard associated with mold exposure is the development of allergy. For people with preexisting asthma, exposure to mold can lead to an increase in the number and frequency of asthma attacks. Despite a large amount of material on the Internet and elsewhere claiming that mold exposure is associ-

TABLE 5.1 – PEDIATRIC ENVIRONMENTAL HOME ASSESSMENT SURVEY

Pediatric Environmental Home Assessment
http://www.healthyhomestraining.org/Nurse/PEHA_Survey.doc

RESIDENT REPORTED INFORMATION
Bolded responses indicate areas of greater concern.

General Housing Characteristics

Type of Ownership	❏ Own house	❏ Market rate rental hsg.	❏ Subsidized rental hsg.	❏ Shelter
Age of Home	❏ **Pre-1950**	❏ **1950-1978**	❏ Post-1978	❏ **Don't know**
Structural Foundation	❏ Basement	❏ Slab on grade	❏ Crawlspace	❏ **Don't know**
Floors Lived In (check all that apply)	❏ Basement	❏ 1st	❏ 2nd	❏ 3rd or higher
Heating — **Fuel Used**	❏ Natural gas / LPG	❏ Oil	❏ Electric	❏ Wood
Heating — **Sources in Home**	❏ Baseboards	❏ Radiators	❏ Forced hot air vents	❏ **Other:** _____
Heating — **Filters Changed**	❏ Yes	❏ **No**	❏ HEPA air filter	❏ **Don't know**
Heating — **Control**	❏ Easy to control heat	❏ Hard to control heat		
Cooling	❏ Windows	❏ Central/window AC	❏ Fans	❏ None
Ventilation (check all that apply)	❏ Open windows	❏ Kitchen/bathroom fans	❏ Central ventilation	

Indoor Pollutants

Mold and Moisture	❏ Use dehumidifier ❏ No damage	❏ **Use vaporizer or humidifier**	❏ **Musty odor evident**	❏ **Visible water / mold damage**
Pets — **Presence**	❏ No pets	❏ Cat #_____	❏ Dog #_____	❏ Other: _____
Pets — **Management**	❏ Kept strictly outdoors	❏ Not allowed in patient's bedroom	❏ **Full access in home**	❏ Sleeping location: _____
Pests — **Cockroaches**	❏ None	❏ **Family reports**	❏ **Family shows evidence**	Present in ❏ kitchen ❏ bedroom ❏ other
Pests — **Mice**	❏ None	❏ **Family reports**	❏ **Family shows evidence**	Present in ❏ kitchen ❏ bedroom ❏ other
Pests — **Rats**	❏ None	❏ **Family reports**	❏ **Family shows evidence**	Present in ❏ kitchen ❏ bedroom ❏ other
Pests — **Bedbugs**	❏ None	❏ **Family reports**	❏ **Family shows evidence**	Present in ❏ bedroom ❏ other

TABLE 5.1—(CONTINUED)

Lead Paint Hazards	❏ Tested and passed	❏ Tested, failed, and mitigated	❏ **Not tested / Don't know**	❏ **Loose, peeling, or chipping paint**
Asbestos	❏ Tested – None present	❏ Tested, failed, and mitigated	❏ **Not tested / Don't know**	❏ **Damaged material**
Radon	❏ Tested and passed	❏ Tested, failed, and mitigated	❏ **Not tested / Don't know**	❏ **Failed test but not mitigated**
Health and Safety Alarms	❏ Smoke alarm working and well placed	❏ CO alarm working and one on each floor	❏ **CO alarm does not log peak level**	❏ **No smoke** ❏ **No CO alarm**
Tobacco Smoke Exposure	❏ No smoking allowed	❏ Smoking allowed outdoors	❏ **Smoking allowed indoors** ❏ **bedroom** ❏ **playroom**	❏ **Total # smokers in household:** _____ ❏ **Mother smokes**
Other Irritants	❏ None	❏ **Air fresheners**	❏ **Potpourri, incense, candles**	❏ **Other strong odors:** _____
Type of Cleaning	❏ Vacuum (non HEPA)	❏ HEPA vacuum	❏ Damp mop and damp dusting	❏ Sweep or dry mop

OBSERVED INFORMATION

Bolded responses indicate areas of greater concern.

Home Environment				
Drinking Water Source	❏ Public water system	❏ **Household Well**		
Kitchen — Cleanliness	❏ No soiling	❏ Trash or garbage sealed	❏ **Trash or garbage not sealed**	❏ **Wall/ceiling/ floor damage**
Kitchen — Ventilation	❏ Functioning stove exhaust fan/vent	❏ **Mold growth present**	❏ **Broken stove exhaust fan/vent**	❏ **No stove exhaust fan/vent**
Bathroom	❏ Functioning exhaust fan/vent/ window	❏ **Mold growth present**	❏ **Needs cleaning and maintenance**	❏ **Wall/ceiling/ floor damage**
Basement	❏ None/No Access	❏ **Mold growth present**	❏ **Needs cleaning and maintenance**	❏ **Wall/ceiling/ floor damage**
Living Room	❏ No soiling	❏ **Mold growth present**	❏ **Needs cleaning and maintenance**	❏ **Wall/ceiling/ floor damage**
Laundry area	❏ None	❏ Well maintained	❏ **Dryer not vented outside**	❏ Hang clothes to dry

TABLE 5.1—(CONTINUED)

Home Safety * can indicate housing code violation			
General			
Active renovation or remodeling	❏ Yes	❏ No	
*Stairs, protective walls, railings, porches	❏ Yes	❏ **No**	
*Hallway lighting	❏ Adequate	❏ **Inadequate**	
Poison control number	❏ Posted by phone	❏ **Not posted by phone**	
Family fire escape plan	❏ Developed and have copy available	❏ **None**	
Electrical appliances (radio, hair dryer, space heater)	❏ Not used near water	❏ **Used near water**	
Matches and lighters stored	❏ Out of child's reach	❏ **Within child's reach**	
Exterior environment	❏ Well maintained	❏ **Abundant trash and debris**	❏ **Chipping, peeling paint**	❏ **Broken window(s)**
Young Children Present	❏ Yes	❏ No	
Coffee, hot liquids, and foods	❏ Out of child's reach	❏ **Within child's reach**	
Cleaning supplies stored	❏ Out of child's reach	❏ **Within child's reach**	
Medicine and vitamins stored	❏ Out of child's reach	❏ **Within child's reach**	
Child (less than six years old) been tested for lead poisoning	❏ Within past 6 months Result: _____	❏ **Within past year or more.** When? _____ Result: _____	❏ No
Child watched by an adult while in the tub	❏ Always	❏ **Most of the time**	❏ No
*Home's hot water temperature	❏ <120 F	❏ **>120 F**	❏ **Don't know**
Non-accordion toddler gates used	❏ At top of stairs	❏ **At bottom of stairs**	❏ No

TABLE 5.1—(CONTINUED)

Crib mattress	❑ Fits well	❑ Loose	❑ NA	
Window guards	❑ Yes	❑ No		
Window blind cords	❑ Split cord	❑ Looped cord		

Sleep Environment				
Patient's sleep area	❑ Own room	❑ Shared # in room_____	❑ Other	
# Beds	❑ 0	❑ 1	❑ 2	❑ More than 2
Allergen impermeable encasings on beds	❑ On mattress and boxspring (zippered)	❑ On mattress only (zippered)	❑ On mattress (not zippered)	❑ No mattress covers
Pillows	❑ Allergen-proof	❑ Washable	❑ Feather/ down	
Bedding	❑ Washable	❑ Wool/not washable	❑ Feather/ down	
Flooring	❑ Hardwood/Tile/ Linoleum	❑ Small area rug	❑ Large area rug	❑ Wall-to-wall carpet
Dust/mold catchers	❑ Stuffed animals/ washable toys ❑ No clutter	❑ Non-washable toys	❑ Plants	❑ Other _____
Window	❑ Washable shades/ curtains	❑ Washable blinds	❑ Curtains/ drapes	❑ No window/ poor ventilation
Other irritants	❑ Abundant cosmetics and fragrances			

Source: With permission from the National Center for Healthy Housing.

ated with brain problems such as inattention, confusion, memory loss, and other symptoms, there is no good scientific evidence to support those claims (Board on Health Promotion and Disease Prevention 2004; Mazur and Kim 2006; Heseltine and Rosen 2009). Mold growth can also result in the release of mycotoxins that can irritate respiratory pathways, including lungs and nasal passages, and result in cough or runny nose symptoms, even outside of allergic pathways.

Asbestos

Asbestos was commonly used decades ago as insulation around boilers and pipes, in ceiling and floor tiles, and other areas. This asbestos may be disturbed and released into the air during renovation or other work. Airborne asbestos may be inhaled into the lung, possibly resulting in mesothelioma or lung cancer years after exposure.

TABLE 5.2—AGENCY FOR TOXIC SUBSTANCES AND DISEASE REGISTRY EXPOSURE HISTORY FORM

Agency for Toxic Substances and Disease Registry
Taking an Exposure History Case Studies in Environmental Medicine (CSEM)

Appendix 1: Exposure History Form

Part 1. Exposure Survey

Name: _____Date:_____

Please circle the appropriate answer. Birth date: _____Sex (circle one): Male Female

1. Are you currently exposed to any of the following?		
metals	no	yes
dust or fibers	no	yes
chemicals	no	yes
fumes	no	yes
radiation	no	yes
loud noise, vibration, extreme heat or cold	no	yes
biologic agents	no	yes
2. Have you been exposed to any of the above in the past?	no	yes
3. Do any household members have contact with metals, dust, fibers, chemicals, fumes, radiation, or biologic agents?	no	yes

If you answered yes to any of the items above, describe your exposure in detail—how you were exposed; to what you were exposed, to what extent (how much) you were exposed if you know. If you need more space, please use a separate sheet of paper.

4. Do you know the names of the metals, dusts, fibers, chemicals, fumes, or radiation that you are/were exposed to? [If yes, list them below.]	no	yes
5. Do you get the material on your skin or clothing?	no	yes
6. Are your work clothes laundered at home?	no	yes
7. Do you shower at work?	no	yes
8. Can you smell the chemical or material you are working with?	no	yes
9. Do you use protective equipment such as gloves, masks, respirator, hearing protectors? [If yes, list the protective equipment used.]	no	yes
10. Have you been advised to use protective equipment?	no	yes

TABLE 5.2—(CONTINUED)

11. Have you been instructed in the use of protective equipment?	no	yes
12. Do you wash your hands with solvents?	no	yes
13. Do you smoke at the workplace?	no	yes
at home?	no	yes
14. Are you exposed to secondhand tobacco smoke at the workplace?	no	yes
at home?	no	yes
15. Do you eat at the workplace?	no	yes
16. Do you know of any coworkers experiencing similar or unusual symptoms?	no	yes
17. Are family members experiencing similar or unusual symptoms?	no	yes
18. Has there been a change in the health or behavior of family pets?	no	yes
19. Do your symptoms seem to be aggravated by a specific activity?	no	yes
20. Do your symptoms get either worse or better at work?	no	yes
at home?	no	yes
on weekends?	no	yes
on vacation?	no	yes
21. Has anything about your job changed in recent months (such as duties, procedures, overtime)?	no	yes
22. Do you use any traditional or alternative medicines?	no	yes
23. Have you or your child ever eaten non-food items, such as paint, plaster, dirt, clay?	no	yes

If you answered yes to any of the questions, please explain.

Part 2. Work History   Name: _____

A. Occupational Profile   Birth date: _____ Sex: Male Female

The following questions refer to your current or most recent job:
Job title: _____Describe this job: _____
Type of industry:_____
Name of employer: _____
Date job began: _____
Are you still working in this job? Yes   No
If no, when did this job end? _____

TABLE 5.2—(CONTINUED)

Fill in the table below listing all jobs you have worked including short-term, seasonal, part-time employment, and military service. Begin with your most recent job. Use additional paper if necessary.

Dates of Employment	Job Title and Description of Work	Exposures*	Protective Equipment

*List the chemicals, dusts, fibers, fumes, radiation, biologic agents (i.e., molds or viruses) and physical agents (i.e., extreme heat, cold, vibration, noise) that you were exposed to at this job.

Have you ever worked at a job or hobby in which you came in contact with any of the following by breathing, touching, or ingesting (swallowing)? If yes, please check the circle beside the name.

○ Acids	○ Chloroprene	○ Methylene chloride	○ Styrene
○ Alcohols (industrial)	○ Chromates	○ Nickel	○ Talc
○ Alkalies	○ Coal dust	○ PBBs	○ TDI or MDI
○ Ammonia	○ Dichlorobenzene	○ PCBs	○ Toluene
○ Arsenic	○ Ethylene dibromide	○ Perchloroethylene	○ Trichloroethylene
○ Asbestos	○ Ethylene dichloride	○ Pesticides	○ Trinitrotoluene
○ Benzene	○ Fiberglass	○ Phenol	○ Vinyl chloride
○ Beryllium	○ Halothane	○ Phosgene	○ Welding fumes
○ Cadmium	○ Isocyanates	○ Radiation	○ X-rays
○ Carbon tetrachloride	○ Ketones	○ Rock dust	○ Other (specify)
○ Chlorinated naphthalenes	○ Lead	○ Silica powder	
○ Chloroform	○ Mercury	○ Solvents	

TABLE 5.2—(CONTINUED)

B. Occupational Exposure Inventory

Please circle the appropriate answer.

1. Have you ever been off work for more than 1 day because of an illness related to work?	no	yes
2. Have you ever been advised to change jobs or work assignments because of any health problems or injuries?	no	yes
3. Has your work routine changed recently?	no	yes
4. Is there poor ventilation in your workplace?	no	yes

Part 3. Environmental History

Please circle the appropriate answer.

1. Do you live next to or near an industrial plant, commercial business, dump site, or nonresidential property?	no	yes
2. Which of the following do you have in your home? Please circle those that apply. Air conditioner Air purifier Central heating (gas or oil?) Gas stove Electric stove Fireplace Wood Humidifier		
3. Have you recently acquired new furniture or carpet, refinished furniture, or remodeled your home?	no	yes
4. Have you weatherized your home recently?	no	yes
5. Are pesticides or herbicides (bug or weed killers; flea and tick sprays, collars, powders, or shampoos) used in your home or garden, or on pets?	no	yes
6. Do you (or any household member) have a hobby or craft?	no	yes
7. Do you work on your car?	no	yes
8. Have you ever changed your residence because of a health problem?	no	yes
9. Does your drinking water come from a private well, city water supply, or grocery store?	no	yes
10. Approximately what year was your home built?_____		
If you answered yes to any of the questions, please explain.		

Source: Developed by the Agency for Toxic Substances and Disease Registry in cooperation with the National Institute for Occupational Safety and Health, 1992.

IS THERE ONGOING OR PLANNED RENOVATION?

Home renovation before the birth of a baby, to update the room decor as the child grows, or to accommodate an elderly relative move is common. Improper renovation procedures may expose residents to lead or other dusts, asbestos, and molds. Newly installed carpets may release irritating or toxic vapors. These exposures may be of particular concern to a pregnant woman, her fetus, or her child.

HAVE CARBON MONOXIDE DETECTORS AND SMOKE ALARMS BEEN INSTALLED?

Unintentional CO poisoning causes hundreds of deaths in the United States each year. CO is a combustion by-product, with the source being heating systems, hot water heaters, or gas stoves. Laws in many states now require CO detectors. Smoke alarms with working lithium batteries allow families up to three minutes to escape a home fire. They should be placed on every level of the home, in every bedroom or sleeping area, and replaced in their entirety once every 10 years.

WHAT TYPE OF HEATING/AIR CONDITIONING SYSTEM DOES THE HOME HAVE?

Wood stoves and fireplaces emit respiratory irritants (nitrogen dioxide, respirable particulates, and polycyclic aromatic hydrocarbons), especially when they are not properly vented and maintained. Gas stoves, which may produce nitrogen dioxide, are used in more than half of U.S. homes. Respiratory symptoms may occur when gas stoves are used for supplemental heat. Wood stoves, fireplaces, and other fuel-burning appliances may be sources of CO.

WHERE AND HOW ARE CHEMICALS AND PESTICIDES STORED?

Pesticides and other chemicals can cause acute poisoning and death, as well as subacute and chronic poisoning. Integrated pest management (U.S. Environmental Protection Agency 2009b) is a preferable approach that uses regular monitoring (rather than regularly scheduled chemical applications) to determine if and when treatments are needed. If toxic chemicals are used, they should be placed out of children's reach. Chemicals should be stored in original containers and never in containers such as soda or juice bottles.

Children may inhale and absorb pesticide residues as they crawl or play on freshly sprayed outdoor surfaces such as lawns and gardens, or on indoor surfaces such as upholstery or rugs. Pesticide residues may adhere to plush toys.

HAS THE HOME BEEN TESTED FOR RADON?

Approximately 10% of lung cancer cases in the United States are attributable to radon. Lung cancer causes approximately 20,000 deaths per year, and radon is a preventable exposure. Radon is a naturally occurring, colorless, odorless gas that is emitted from the ground on which the building is constructed (Gray et al. 2009). An estimated 8 million homes have elevated levels of radon, defined as levels greater than 4 pci/L. Indoor radon levels vary by state and region of the country and therefore must be checked in each domicile. Sample collection is done with a simple, passive device that is left in the basement for a specified period of time and mailed to a laboratory for analysis or with an active air sampling system that collects data for 24–48 hours and that is then studied in a laboratory. Testing is generally inexpensive. If levels of radon are elevated in a home, it is best to create an active radon mitigation system to disperse the gas outdoors and away from indoor exposure.

PHYSICAL EXAMINATION

The physical examination of an individual being evaluated for a possible housing-related medical problem would be exactly the same as for any other individual. There are no specific stigmata or pathognomonic findings associated with most housing-related exposures. For example, an individual who has asthma related to exposure to rodent or cockroach antigen in a home will have the same physical findings as an individual who has asthma related to ragweed pollen.

LABORATORY TESTING

The utility of measuring toxicants in patients, particularly of toxic chemicals, is more limited than one would think. There are some major categories to focus on:

heavy metals (e.g., lead and mercury), pesticides, and environmental tobacco smoke. Laboratory evaluation of an environmental health issue, as in other clinical settings, should be driven by clinical symptomatology or known exposures. Biological samples sent for large numbers of tests (e.g., environmental health screening panels) are more likely to result in false positives than true positives. Tests should be done to confirm suspected exposures, not as screening tests to look for unknown exposures (Hoffman, Buka, and Philips 2007). In particular, hair testing, except in research settings, is unreliable and should not be used for the clinical evaluation of patients with suspected environmentally related problems (Barrett 1985; Eastern Research Group 2001; Frisch and Schwartz 2002; Harkins and Susten 2003; Klevay et al. 1987; Seidel et al. 2001; Wennig 2000; Yoshinaga et al. 1990).

Exposure to Heavy Metals

A simple serum test can show whether there is lead in the blood. A blood lead level greater than 10 µg/dL is defined by the CDC as a level of concern; however, it is well recognized by the CDC and others that blood lead levels less than 10 µg/dL are potentially injurious to a child's health (Canfield et al. 2003). Serum samples should be obtained by venipuncture when possible. In the acute setting of a lead elevation greater than 30 µg/dL, an abdominal x-ray can be used to determine whether radio-opaque material consistent with a chip of lead-containing paint is in the stomach or intestines.

Mercury exposures in the home setting can occur when a broken mercury thermometer is cleaned up improperly, when students remove mercury from a school laboratory and spread it in the home, or when mercury is used for religious purposes (Baughman 2006; Riley et al. 2001). Mercury concentrations can be measured in urine, ideally with a 24-hour collection; however, it is important to restrict seafood intake for 3 days before the collection, and it may also be important to separate the mercury found in the urine into organic and inorganic components. This is referred to as speciating the mercury. Toxicity is correlated with the inorganic component. Mercury levels from 10 to 20 µg/L are evidence of excessive exposure, and neurologic signs may be present at values greater than 100 µg/L. However, urinary mercury concentration does not necessarily correlate with chronicity or severity of toxic effects, especially if the mercury exposure has been intermittent or variable in intensity. With exposure to metallic mercury, whole blood mercury concentration can be tested, but values tend to return to normal within 1–2 days after the exposure. Measuring mercury in urine after administration of a chelating agent and measuring mercury in the serum are not reliable. All urine testing should be done using an accredited laboratory or one associated with a state department of environment or public health.

Exposure to Environmental Tobacco Smoke

It is generally thought that a history of presence of smokers in the home is a good marker for clinical exposure. Maternal reports of smoke exposure correlate well with biological markers, although it is stronger among mothers who smoke than among mothers who do not smoke but have smokers in the home. In experimental settings, cotinine, the by-product of nicotine exposure, can be measured in serum, urine, and saliva, although these are more widely used in research than clinical settings.

ALLERGY TESTING

Several mechanisms are available to test for allergy to environmental health hazards, such as dust mites and various danders, that a patient can be exposed to in a home setting. A review of the utility of skin testing and the use of radio-absorbent allergen testing is beyond the scope of this chapter (Bernstein et al. 2008). Most clinicians will test patients to see whether they are allergic to an exposure if they determine by history taking that it is present in the home first.

LABORATORY EVALUATION OF INDIVIDUALS WITH DEVELOPMENTAL DISABILITIES

The clinical and laboratory evaluation of individuals with developmental disabilities for possible environmental etiologies of their problems is described by Hussain et al. (2007). Laboratory testing of children for an environmental toxicant as the etiology of developmental delay is almost never indicated. Although elevated blood levels are not etiologically related to delay in children with developmental disabilities, these children may have elevated blood lead levels at an older age than normally developing children because of their persistent hand-to-mouth activities (Shannon and Graef 1996). This makes blood lead testing in children with persistent hand-to-mouth activities more reasonable at older ages than in other children.

TESTING IN THE ENVIRONMENT

Unfortunately, in many instances, testing the home environment for sources of exposure to environmental hazards does not prove to be clinically useful. A detailed history is often the best indicator of exposure.

Testing in the environment depends on which substance is suspected. Testing for lead in paint or dust in the home should be done by a certified lead specialist. Testing for lead chips in outside soil or testing of water should be done by state departments of public health. If there was a spill of a relatively large quantity (e.g., several ounces) of metallic mercury after clean-up, evaluation of air levels of mercury with a Jerome meter can be useful to determine if it is safe for people to return to the environment. Pesticide residue testing can be done on soil or ground water, although this should be done only by a state public health laboratory. Environmental tobacco smoke testing can be done through passive diffusion monitors, but this is more useful in the research setting given the costs and accuracy of biomarkers in children.

Allergen Sampling

Allergen sampling is commonly used in research settings and less used in clinical settings to determine exposures in the homes.

Mold Sampling

Given the thousands of molds that exist, mold sampling can be expensive and is not commonly useful in clinical settings (Committee on Damp Indoor Spaces and Health 2004; Heseltine and Rosen 2009). A good visual inspection of a home can show signs of dampness, water damage, and mold growth. The nose is very sensitive to the odor of mold (or mildew, which is the same thing) and an extremely reliable indicator of mold growth. Measuring indoor humidity with a humidistat is easy and may be useful.

Well Water Sampling

Up to one in five U.S. families obtain their drinking water from private wells that are not regulated by the U.S. Environmental Protection Agency. State and local regulation is variable, but generally minimal. Wells can be contaminated with microbes, fertilizers, pesticides, lead, arsenic, chromium VI, radon, fluoride, volatile organic compounds, uranium, radon, methyl tertiary butyl ether, perchlorate, and other chemicals. New wells, or the well in any home that is new to a family, should be tested for coliform bacteria, nitrates, inorganic chemicals (total dissolved solids, iron, magnesium, calcium, chloride), fluoride, radon, and lead. Thereafter, wells should be tested at least annually for coliforms and nitrates. Additional testing may be indicated in the following special situations: (1) There is a pregnant or nursing woman in the home; (2) there are unexplained illnesses in the household; (3) a dangerous contaminant is found in a well in close proximity; (4) there is a change in the appearance, odor, or taste of the well water; (5) there is a chemical spill in proximity of the well; or (6) there was a significant repair or replacement in the well (Rogan and Brady 2009). Nitrate levels should be less than 3 mg/L. Other test results should be interpreted in conjunction with the local health department.

EXAMPLES OF PATIENTS WITH BUILDING-RELATED ISSUES

Case 1: Adult

A 57-year-old woman who had taught fifth grade for 20 years presented in the fall with a 6-year history of cough, which would be fine in the fall and winter but generally worsen during the spring. The cough would then clear in the summer when she moved to her summer home at the beach. She had been treated for asthma over the preceding 18 months with oral and inhaled steroids and inhaled bronchodilators. She also had been treated with allergy immunotherapy shots. Her medical history included pneumonia at age 32 years and 10 years of cigarette use before quitting 20 years before presentation. No rashes, allergic rhinitis, or headaches were noted.

Physical examination results were normal and included normal pulmonary examination results. However, spirometry testing from spring to summer reflected a 20% improvement in both forced vital capacity and forced expiratory volume in 1 second after she vacated the home.

The elementary school where she taught had no history of poor air quality. Because of the chronology and the fact that she was fine in the school building for much of the school year, the first environment to investigate was the home.

The home inspection showed the first-floor bedroom where she slept had a moldy smell. There was a leaky skylight in the bathroom attached to the bedroom and a mulch pile outside the bedroom window sloped toward the house with pooling water up against the bedroom wall.

After an addition was put on the house six years ago, each spring, with much rainfall, the roof around the skylight would leak into the house, wetting the wall-to-wall carpet and causing mold growth. Moreover, the landscaping outside the house was also allowing water to pool into the walls, causing potential water intrusion and mold growth. The family had the roof replaced and skylight sealed to avoid leaks, pulled up the wall-to-wall carpet and replaced it with smooth flooring, and regraded the outside landscaping away from the house to avoid pooling water. Her symptoms resolved, and lung function returned to normal.

Case 2: Child

Sarah and David bring their 3-year-old son Jose in for a yearly physical examination. Sarah is 6 months pregnant, and the family will be moving from a fifth-floor apartment to a house before the baby is born. The house has a playroom in the basement that the family plans to use extensively and a bedroom in the basement that they may use for Jose when he gets older.

This situation could play out in two ways in a clinical setting. First, the parents could ask what they need to think about before they move into this new home. The best response on the part of the clinician would be to educate the family about the potential for radon exposure, the level of concern for radon (>4 pCi/L of air), how to test for radon levels in the basement, and a simple means of mitigating the radon exposure if the level is high (U.S. Environmental Protection Agency 2009a). The clinician could also educate the family about the importance of keeping the basement dry, for instance, with a dehumidifier and avoiding carpet in this potentially damp area.

In the alternative scenario, the parents would not even know to ask about the housing environment in the context of the health of the children. Then it would be up to the clinician to ask if the family has thought about the potential problem of radon in the basement of the home. If the family knows what to do, the clinician merely needs to provide positive feedback. If the family does not know what to do, then the clinician can proceed as described.

RESOURCES FOR THE PRACTITIONER

Government Resources

Local, state, and federal agency offices can serve as resources for patients and practitioners. Each municipality or county has a local board of health. This may consist of only a few people and a volunteer board in small towns or of hundreds of workers with many divisions in large cities. These boards of health enforce both local and state codes for housing, commonly referred to as "sanitary codes," and are important to investigate, particularly if a patient is renting and will require a landlord to make changes to a house for health reasons. States often have Departments of Public Health that generally have environmental health divisions, usually around toxins such as lead or radon, but many are adopting healthy homes divisions that can be helpful. Some cities, counties, and states now have Departments of the Environment that are separate from their Departments of Health. It may be necessary to check which agency has jurisdiction over which type of housing-related environmental health problem. Each region of the country has federal offices of the Environmental Protection Agency, Department of Housing and Urban Development, and Department of Health and Human Services, which can also serve as resources for information or investigation.

NON-GOVERNMENT RESOURCES

Pediatric Environmental Health Specialty Units

There are ten Pediatric Environmental Health Specialty Units (PEHSUs) in the United States, one PEHSU in Canada, and one PEHSU in Mexico (Table 5.3). The PEHSUs have two goals: 1) to provide education to health professionals and others about children's environmental health and 2) to provide consultations to health professionals and others regarding children's environmental health issues. Practitioners or others seeking information about housing-related health issues in children should contact their regional PEHSU. All of the PEHSUs have an adult-trained occupational environmental health physician as part of the core team. Therefore, PEHSUs can also be a resource where exposures involve adults in a family as well as children (Paulson et al. 2009). PEHSUs are organized to deal with long-term, low-dose exposures or the long-term sequela of acute exposures. Poison-control centers should be relied on for assistance in management of acute intoxications.

Association of Occupational and Environmental Clinics

The clinics that are part of the Association of Occupational and Environmental Clinics are a resource for information and referrals of adults with housing-related medical problems. The 60 affiliated clinics are independent of industry and equipped to provide consultation on adults. A list of clinics is available at the Association of Occupational and Environmental Clinics Website (http://www.aoec.org).

Poison-Control Centers

Poison-control centers (national toll-free number 1-800-222-1222) are the essential resource for consultations about children or adults with acute ingestions or exposures to household or other environmental health hazards. This includes pesticides, household cleaning supplies, and other products. If a person is having a seizure, not breathing, or unconscious, others should call 911.

Online Resources

There are numerous online resources available for information about housing-related environmental health issues (Table 5.4).

Working with Other Health Professionals

The evaluation of a building-related health symptom should be a multidisciplinary task with various health professionals partnering for mutual assistance. For example, industrial hygienists, who are often certified by the American Industrial Hygienist Asso-

TABLE 5.3 — NORTH AMERICAN PEDIATRIC ENVIRONMENTAL HEALTH SPECIALTY UNITS, BY COUNTRY/REGION

EPA Region I: CT, MA, ME, NH, RI, VT
New England Pediatric Environmental Health Specialty Unit
http://www.childrenshospital.org/pehc
Boston, MA
Toll Free: 1-888-CHILD14 (1-888-244-5314)

EPA Region II: NJ, NY, PR, VI
Mount Sinai Pediatric Environmental Health Specialty Unit
http://www.mssm.edu/cpm/pehsu
New York, NY
Toll Free: 1-866-265-6201
Phone: (212) 241-5756

EPA Region III: DE, DC, MD, PA, VA, WV
Mid-Atlantic Center for Children's Health and the Environment
http://www.health-e-kids.org
Washington DC
Toll Free: 1-866-622-2431
Phone: (202) 471-4829

EPA Region IV: AL, FL, GA, KY, MS, NC, SC, TN
The Southeast Pediatric Environmental Health Specialty Unit
http://www.sph.emory.edu/PEHSU
Atlanta, GA
Toll Free: 877-33PEHSU (1-877-337-3478)
Phone: (404) 727-9428

EPA Region V: IL, IN, MI, MN, OH, WI
Great Lakes Center for Children's Environmental Health
http://www.uic.edu/sph/glakes/kids
Chicago, IL
Toll Free (866) 967-7337
Phone: (312) 864-5526

EPA Region VI: AR, LA, NM, OK, TX
Southwest Center for Pediatric Environmental Health
http://www.swcpeh.org
Tyler, TX
Toll-free: (888) 901-5665 (AR, LA, NM, OK, and TX only)
Phone: (903) 877-5884

TABLE 5.3—(CONTINUED)

EPA Region VII: IA, KS, MO, NE
MidAmerica Pediatric Environmental Health Specialty Unit
http://www.childrensmercy.org/mapehsu
Kansas City, KS
Toll Free: 1-800-421-9916
Phone: (913) 588-6638

EPA Region VIII: CO, MT, ND, SD, UT, WY
Rocky Mountain Regional Pediatric Environmental Health Specialty Unit
http://www.rmrpehsu.org
Denver, CO
Toll Free: (877) 800-5554

EPA Region IX: AZ, CA, HI, NV
Pediatric Environmental Health Specialty Unit
http://www.ucsf.edu/ucpehsu
866-UC-PEHSU (1-866-827-3478) (same toll-free phone for both sites - San Francisco and Irvine)
San Francisco Phone: (415) 206-4083
Irvine Phone: (949) 824-1857

EPA Region X: AK, ID, OR, WA
Northwest Pediatric Environmental Health Specialty Unit
http://www.depts.washington.edu/pehsu
Seattle, WA
Toll Free West of the Mississippi River: 1-877-KID-CHEM (1-877-543-2436)
Phone: (206) 744-9380

Canada
Pediatric Environmental Health Clinic
http://www.albertahealthservices.ca/services.asp?pid=serviceandrid=5903
Edmonton, AB, Canada
Phone: (780) 735-2443 (local and outside of Canada)

Mexico
Unidad Pediatrica Ambiental - Mexico Pediatric Environmental Health Specialty Unit
http://www.upa-pehsu.org
Cuernavaca, Mexico
Phone: 01-800-001-7777 (Inside Mexico)
Phone: 52-777-102-1259 (Outside Mexico)

TABLE 5.4 – RESOURCES FOR HOUSING-RELATED ENVIRONMENTAL HEALTH INFORMATION

Organization	Contact Information
Government	
Agency for Toxic Substances and Disease Registry (ATSDR) Department of Health and Human Services 1600 Clifton Rd NE; Mail Stop E-28 Atlanta, GA 30333	Web: http://www.atsdr.cdc.gov Information Center Clearinghouse: Phone: 404-639-6360 Fax: 404-639-0744 Emergency Response Branch Phone: 404-639-0615
ATSDR Toxicological Profiles	Web: http://www.atsdr.cdc.gov/toxpro2.html
ATSDR Regional Offices	Web: http://www.atsdr.cdc.gov/oro_contact.html
Consumer Product Safety Commission 4340 East West Hwy Bethesda, MD 20814	Web: http://www.cpsc.gov Phone: 800-638-2772 Fax: 301-504-0124
Department of Housing and Urban Development Office of Healthy Homes and Lead Hazard Control 451 7th St SW Washington, DC 20410	Web: http://www.hud.gov/offices/lead
Environmental Protection Agency (EPA) 1200 Pennsylvania Ave NW Washington, DC 20460	Web: http://www.epa.gov Phone: 202-272-0167
EPA Office of Children's Health Protection	Web: yosemite.epa.gov/ochp/ochpweb.nsf/homepage Office of Child Health Protection Phone: 202-564-2188
EPA Office of Pesticide Programs	Web: http://www.epa.gov/pesticides Office of Pesticide Programs Phone: 703-305-5017 National Pesticides Hotline: 800-222-1222
EPA Office of Air and Radiation	Office main Web: http://www.epa.gov/oar Indoor air Web: http://www.epa.gov/iaq Indoor Air Quality Information Clearinghouse Phone: 800-438-4318
EPA Office of Pollution Prevention and Toxics	Web: http://www.epa.gov/opptintr/index.html Toxic Substances Control Act (TSCA) Information Line: 202-554-1404

TABLE 5.4 – (CONTINUED)

Organization	Contact Information
National Center for Environmental Health (NCEH) Centers for Disease Control and Prevention 4770 Buford Hwy, NE Mail Stop F-28 Atlanta, GA 30341-3724	Web: http://www.cdc.gov/nceh E-mail: ncehinfo@cdc.gov NCEH Health Line: 888-232-6789
NCEH Asthma Program	Web: http://www.cdc.gov/nceh/airpollution/asthma
NCEH Lead Poisoning Prevention Program	Web: http://www.cdc.gov/nceh/lead/lead.htm
NCEH Healthy Home Initiative	Web: http://www.cdc.gov/nceh/lead/healthyhomes.htm
National Library of Medicine, Environmental Health, and Toxicology	Web: sis.nlm.nih.gov/enviro.html
TOXNET	Web: toxnet.nlm.nih.gov
ToxMystery (web game for children 7-11 years old about household chemical hazards)	Web: toxmystery.nlm.nih.gov/
Nongovernmental Organizations	
Allergy and Asthma Network Mothers of Asthmatics 2751 Prosperity Ave, Suite 150 Fairfax, VA 22031	Web: http://www.aanma.org Phone: 800-878-4403 Fax: 703-573-7794
American Cancer Society 1599 Clifton Rd NE Atlanta, GA 30329	Web: http://www.cancer.org Phone: 404-320-3333 or 800-ACS-2345 Fax: 404-329-7530
American Lung Association 61 Broadway 6th Floor New York, NY 10016	Web: http://www.lungusa.org Phone: 800-LUNG-USA
American Public Health Association 800 I St NW Washington, DC 20001	Web: http://www.apha.org Phone: 202-777-2742
Asthma and Allergy Foundation of America 1233 20th St NW Suite 402 Washington, DC 20005	Web: http://www.aafa.org Phone: 202-466-7643 Fax: 202-466-8940
Beyond Pesticides 701 E St SE, #200 Washington DC 20003	Web: http://www.beyondpesticides.org/main.html Phone: 202-543-5450 Fax: 202-543-4791
Children's Health Environmental Coalition PO Box 1540 Princeton, NJ 08542	Web: http://www.checnet.org

TABLE 5.4 – (CONTINUED)

Earth Portal	Web: http://www.earthportal.org/
Encyclopedia of the Earth	Web: http://www.eoearth.org/
Environmental Defense 257 Park Ave S New York, NY 10010	Web: http://www.environmentaldefense.org Phone: 212-505-2100 Fax: 212-505-2375
Environmental Justice Resource Center at Clark Atlanta University 223 James P Brawley Dr SW Atlanta, GA 30314	Web: http://www.ejrc.cau.edu Phone: 404-880-6911 Fax: 404-880-6909
Environmental Working Group 1436 U St NW Suite 100 Washington, DC 20009	Web: http://www.ewg.org
Home Safety Council 1250 Eye Street, NW, Suite 1000 Washington, DC 20005	http://www.homesafetycouncil.org
*Home*A*Syst Program* 303 Hiram Smith Hall 1545 Observatory Dr Madison, WI 53706	Web: http://www.uwex.edu/homeasyst Phone: 608-262-0024 Fax: 608-265-2775
National Center for Healthy Housing 10227 Wincopin Circle, Suite 100 Columbia, MD 21044	Web: http://www.centerforhealthyhousing.org/ index. htm Phone: 410-992-0712 Fax: 410-715-2310
National Lead Information Center 422 S Clinton Ave Rochester, NY 14620	Web: http://www.epa.gov/lead/nlic.htm Phone: 800-424-LEAD (5323)
National Pesticide Information Center	Web: http://npic.orst.edu
National Safety Council Environmental Health Center, Indoor Air	Web: http://www.nsc.org/ehc/indoor/wctoc.htm
National Safety Council, Environmental Health Center 1025 Connecticut Ave NW; Suite 1200 Washington, DC 20036	Web: http://www.nsc.org/ehc.htm
Pediatric Environmental Health Specialty Units (PEHSUs)	Web: http://www.aoec.org/pesu.htm http://www.pehsu.net (includes links to all PEHSUs)
World Health Organization Public Health and Environment	Web: http://www.who.int/phe/en

ciation, can partner with primary care providers. Building inspectors can be another partner. Visiting nurses and community health workers are also important visitors in the home setting. Some training exists online for nurses at http://www.nchh.org (Table 5.1).

CONCLUSION

The home environment has a major impact on the health of its inhabitants and visitors. Health care providers can apply many of the same tools that they are already comfortable with—history taking (with additional details related to the home), physical examination (no special activities required), and laboratory evaluation (only a limited array of testing of the individual or the environment makes sense)—in evaluating a patient with a symptom related to the home environment. The use of additional specialists, such as industrial hygienists and visiting nurses, can be helpful. There are numerous Web-based sources of information that a practitioner can use in these evaluations.

REFERENCES

Agency for Toxic Substances and Disease Registry. *Case Studies in Environmental Medicine: Taking an Exposure History.* 2008a. Available at: http://www.atsdr.cdc.gov/csem/exphistory/docs/exposure_history.pdf. Accessed September 15, 2009.

——. *Pediatric Environmental Health Training Module.* 2008b. Available at: http://www.atsdr.cdc.gov/emes/health_professionals/pediatrics.html. Accessed September 14, 2009.

American Academy of Pediatrics Committee on Environmental Health. Chapter 4: How to take an environmental history; Chapter 5: How to do a home inventory of environmental hazards. In: Etzel, R.A., and S.J. Balk, eds. *Pediatric Environmental Health.* 2nd ed. Elk Grove Village, IL: American Academy of Pediatrics, 2006:37–46; 47–50.

Barrett, S. Commercial hair analysis. Science or scam? *JAMA* (1985):254:1041–5.

Baughman, T.A. Elemental mercury spills. *Environ Health Perspect* (2006):114:147–52.

Bernstein, I.L., J.T. Li, D.I. Bernstein, et al.; American Academy of Allergy, Asthma and Immunology; American College of Allergy, Asthma and Immunology. Allergy diagnostic testing: An updated practice parameter. *Ann Allergy Asthma Immunol* (2008):100(Suppl 3):S1–148.

Blatt, J., L. Van Le, T. Weiner, and S. Sailer. Ovarian carcinoma in an adolescent with transgenerational exposure to diethylstilbestrol. *J Pediatr Hematol Oncol* (2003):25:635–6.

Board on Health Promotion and Disease Prevention. *Damp Indoor Spaces and Health.* Institute of Medicine. Washington, DC: National Academies Press, 2004. Available at: http://www.nap.edu/openbook.php?record_id=11011&page=R1. Accessed November 10, 2009.

Brouwers, M.M., W.F. Feitz, L.A. Roelofs, et al. Hypospadias: A transgenerational effect of diethylstilbestrol? *Hum Reprod* (2006):21:666–9.

Canfield, R.L., C.R. Henderson Jr., D.A. Cory-Slechta, C. Cox, T.A. Jusko, and B.P. Lanphear. 2003. Intellectual impairment in children with blood lead concentrations below 10 microg per deciliter. *N Engl J Med* (2003):348:1517–26.

Centers for Disease Control and Prevention. Hypothermia prevention. *MMWR Morb Mortal Wkly Rep* (1988):37:780–2.

Committee on Damp Indoor Spaces and Health. *Damp Indoor Spaces and Health*. Washington, DC: National Academies Press, 2004. Available at: http://www.nap.edu/catalog.php?record_id=11011. Accessed December 14, 2009.

Eastern Research Group. *Hair Analysis Panel Discussion: Exploring the State of the Science* (2001). Available at: http://www.atsdr.cdc.gov/HAC/hair_analysis. Accessed November 9, 2009.

Etzel, R.A., and S.J. Balk, eds. *Pediatric Environmental Health*. 2nd ed. Elk Grove Village, IL: American Academy of Pediatrics, 2006.

Federal Interagency Forum on Aging-Related Statistics. *Older Americans 2006 Update: Key Indicators of Well-Being*. Washington, DC: Federal Interagency Forum on Aging-Related Statistics, 2006.

Frisch, M., and B.S. Schwartz. The pitfalls of hair analysis for toxicants in clinical practice: Three case reports. *Environ Health Perspect* (2002):110:433–6.

Fullilove, M.T. Links between the social and physical environments. *Pediatr Clin N Am* (2001):48:1253–66.

Gee, G.C., and D.C. Payne-Sturges. Environmental health disparities: A framework integrating psychosocial and environmental concepts. *Environ Health Perspect* (2004):112:1645–53.

Golant, S.M. Low-income elderly homeowners in very old dwellings: The need for public policy debate. *J Aging Soc Policy* (2008):20:1–28.

Goldman, R., M. Shannon, and A. Woolf. *Approach to the Environmental Health History* (1999). Available at: http://www.aoec.org/PedEnvHistoryPP4.ppt#256,1,Pediatric Environmental Health. Accessed September 15, 2009.

Gray, A., S. Read, P. McGale, and S. Darby. Lung cancer deaths from indoor radon and the cost effectiveness and potential of policies to reduce them. *BMJ* (2009):338:a3110.

Hansen, D.A. Paternal environmental exposures and gene expression during spermatogenesis: Research review to research framework. *Birth Defects Res C* (2008):84:155–63.

Harkins, D.K., and A.S. Susten. Hair analysis: Exploring the state of the science. *Environ Health Perspect* (2003):111:576–8.

Heseltine, E., and J. Rosen, eds. *WHO Guidelines for Indoor Air Quality, Dampness and Mould*. WHO Regional Office for Europe (2009). Available at: http://www.euro.who.int/document/E92645.pdf. Accessed December 14, 2009.

Hoffman, H.E., I. Buka, and S. Phillips. Medical laboratory investigation of children's environmental health. *Pediatr Clin North Am* (2007):54:399–415.

Hood, E. Dwelling disparities: How poor housing leads to poor health. *Environ Health Perspect* (2005):113:A310–17.

Hughes, M.E., L.J. Waite, T.A. LaPierre, and Y. Luo. All in the family: The impact of caring for grandchildren on grandparents' health. *J Gerontol B Psychol Sci Soc Sci* (2007):62:S108–19.

Hussain, J., A.D. Woolf, M. Sandel, and M.W. Shannon. Environmental evaluation of a child with developmental disability. *Pediatr Clin North Am* (2007):54:47–62.

Joint Center for Housing Studies of Harvard University. *Measuring the Benefits of Home Remodeling.* Cambridge, MA: Joint Center for Housing Studies of Harvard University, 2003.

Kao, H., R. Conant, T. Soriano, and W. McCormick. The past, present, and future of house calls. *Clin Geriatr Med* (2009):25:19–34.

Klevay, L.M., B.R. Bistrian, C.R. Fleming, and C.G. Neumann. Hair analysis in clinical and experimental medicine. *Am J Clin Nutr* (1987):46:233–6.

Makri, A., M. Goveia, J. Balbus, and R. Parkin. Children's susceptibility to chemicals: A review by developmental stage. *J Toxicol Environ Health B Crit Rev* (2004):7:417–35.

Mazur, L.J., and J. Kim; Committee on Environmental Health, American Academy of Pediatrics. Spectrum of noninfectious health effects from molds. *Pediatrics* 2006:118:e1909–26. Review. Erratum in: *Pediatrics* (2007):119:868.

Moya, J., C.F. Bearer, and R.A. Etzel. Children's behavior and physiology and how it affects exposure to environmental contaminants. *Pediatrics* (2004):113:996–1006.

National Academy of Sciences. *Pesticides in the Diets of Infants and Children* (1993). Available at: http://www.nap.edu/catalog.php?record_id=2126. Accessed September 10, 2009.

National Center for Healthy Housing. *Pediatric Environmental Home Assessment On-Line Training for Public Health and Visiting Nurses.* Available at: http://www.healthyhomestraining. org/Nurse/PEHA_Start.htm. Accessed September 15, 2009.

Newbold, R.R, R.B. Hanson, W.N. Jefferson, B.C. Bullock, J. Haseman, and J. A. McLachlan. Increased tumors but uncompromised fertility in the female descendants of mice exposed developmentally to diethylstilbestrol. *Carcinogenesis* (1998):19:1655–63.

——. Proliferative lesions and reproductive tract tumors in male descendants of mice exposed developmentally to diethylstilbestrol. *Carcinogenesis* (2000):21:1355–63.

Newman, S. The living conditions of elderly Americans. *Gerontologist* (2003):43:99–109.

Paulson, J.A., C.J. Karr, J.M. Seltzer, et al. Development of the pediatric environmental health specialty unit network: The North American Experience. *Am J Public Health* (2009):99:S511–16.

Payne-Sturges, D., and G.C. Gee. National environmental health measures for minority and low-income populations: Tracking social disparities in environmental health. *Environ Res* (2006):102:154–71.

Payne-Sturges, D., G.C. Gee, K. Crowder, et al. Workshop summary: Connecting social and environmental factors to measure and track environmental health disparities. *Environ Res* (2006):102:146–53.

Pollack, S.H. Adolescent occupational exposures and pediatric-adolescent take-home exposures. *Pediatr Clin North Am* (2001):48:1267–89.

Riley, D.M., C.A. Newby, T.O. Leal-Almeraz, and V.M. Thomas. Assessing elemental mercury vapor exposure from cultural and religious practices. *Environ Health Perspect* (2001):109:779–84.

Rogan, W.J., and M.T. Brady; Committee on Environmental Health; Committee on Infectious Diseases. Drinking water from private wells and risks to children. *Pediatrics* (2009):123(6):e1123–37.

Seidel, S., R. Kreutzer, D. Smith, S. McNeel, and D. Gilliss. Assessment of commercial laboratories performing hair mineral analysis. *JAMA* (2001):285:67–72 .

Selevan, S. G., C.A. Kimmel, and P. Mendola. Identifying critical windows of exposure for children's health. *Environ Health Perspect* (2000):108(Suppl 3):451–5.

Shannon, M., and J.W. Graef. Lead intoxication in children with pervasive developmental disorders. *J Toxicol Clin Toxicol* (1996):34:177–81.

Stevens, J.A., K.A. Mack, L.J. Paulozzi, and M.F. Ballesteros. Self-reported falls and fall-related injuries among persons aged ≥65 years—United States, 2006. *MMWR Morb Mortal Wkly Rep* (2008):57:225–9.

Thundiyil, J.G., G.M. Solomon, and M.D. Miller. Transgenerational exposures: Persistent chemical pollutants in the environment and breast milk. *Pediatr Clin North Am* (2007):54; 81–101.

U.S. Department of Health and Human Services. *The Surgeon General's Call to Action to Promote Healthy Homes*. Washington, DC: U.S. Department of Health and Human Services, Office of the Surgeon General, 2009.

U.S. Environmental Protection Agency. *A Citizen's Guide to Radon*. 2009a. Available at: http://www.epa.gov/radon/pubs/citguide.html#overview. Accessed March 2, 2010.

——. *Integrated Pest Management (IPM) Principles*. 2009b. Available at: http://www.epa.gov/opp00001/factsheets/ipm.htm. Accessed December 30, 2009.

Viegi, G., M. Simoni, A. Scognamiglio, et al. Indoor air pollution and airway disease. *Int J Tuberc Lung Dis* (2004):8:1401–15.

Weiss, B., and P.J. Landrigan. The developing brain and the environment: An introduction. *Environ Health Perspect* (2000):108:(Suppl 3):373–4.

Wennig, R. Potential problems with the interpretation of hair analysis results. *Forensic Sci Int* (2000):107:5–12.

Wigle, D.T., T.E. Arbuckle, M. Walker, M.G. Wade, S. Liu, and D. Krewski. Environmental hazards: Evidence for effects on child health. *J Toxicol Environ Health B Crit Rev* (2007):10:3–39.

Woodruff, T.J., A. Carlson, J.M. Schwartz, and L.C. Giudice. Proceedings of the Summit on Environmental Challenges to Reproductive Health and Fertility: Executive summary. *Fertil Steril* (2008):89:281–300.

Yoshinaga, J., H. Imai, M. Nakazawa, T. Suzuki, and M. Morita. Lack of significantly positive correlations between elemental concentrations in hair and in organs. *Sci Total Environ* (1990):99:125–35.

Ziegler, E.E., B.B. Edwards, R.L. Jensen, K.R. Mahaffey, and S.J. Fomon. Absorption and retention of lead by infants. *Pediatr Res* (1978):12:29–34.

The Healthy Housing Workforce: Development and Scope of Practice

Mary Jean Brown, ScD, RN,
Charles Treser, MPH, DAAS, and
David Jacobs, PhD, CIH

Over the past century, the once widely recognized connection between the housing profession and the public health profession has atrophied. Although many housing and health professionals once attended joint conferences, had similar academic backgrounds, and even sometimes worked for single local government bodies that integrated housing and health disciplines into one agency, modern specialization has isolated the two.

The connections between housing and health have been understood since antiquity. Standards for building construction date back approximately 4,000 years. The Babylonian King Hammurabi[1] (1792–1750 B.C.E.) (LookLex Encyclopedia 2009) is credited with codifying the laws of the time. The laws addressed the responsibility of the home builder to "construct a quality home and outlined the implications to the builder if injury or harm came to the owner as a result of the failure to do so" (Centers for Disease Control and Prevention [CDC] and U.S. Department of Housing and Urban Development [HUD] 2006). In 1946, the American Public Health Association's Committee on the Hygiene of Housing reprinted *The Basic Principles of Healthful Housing*. The report consists of 30 basic principles with specific requirements and suggested methods of attainment for each. The principles and specific requirements are believed to be the fundamental minimum required for the promotion of physical, mental, and social health, essential in low- and high-cost housing, on the farm and for city dwellers. This report grouped the

---

1 Estimates of the date of emergence of the state of Babylonia correspond with the rise of Hammurabi, even though he was actually the sixth king in his dynasty. Other time reconstructions suggest that he governed around 1728–1686 B.C.E.

30 principles into 4 sets of fundamental needs that housing must satisfy: physiological needs, psychological needs, protection against contagion, and protection against accidents. Even today, these basic principles of healthful housing remain a valuable guide to the design, construction, use, and maintenance of housing units (CDC and HUD 2006).

Unfortunately, in many communities, increased specialization resulting from different funding streams, legal mandates, and organizational efficiencies has separated housing programs from the public health agency. Indeed, even within many public health agencies there is often a gulf between the environmental public health workforce (i.e., the traditional sanitarian or environmental health specialist) and personal health workforce (i.e., the public health nurse or community health worker). Although specialization is a necessity in our modern society, one effect is that housing and health groups may have little knowledge or understanding of the other and fail to recognize the mutual benefits of collaboration. For example, a housing program in Bradford, England, found that health workers by and large did not seem to see anything to do with housing as part of their job, and housing workers were seen as solely interested in the housing structure and the costs of repairs (Allen 2005). Indeed, many public health and housing disciplines have been further subdivided. For example, in major metropolitan areas, the traditional housing code inspector has been replaced by a series of more specialized personnel, such as environmental engineers or building scientists. Current practice in the United States is to address environmental diseases and the housing conditions that cause them on an issue-by-issue basis. A recent structured review showed that 92% of housing interventions published in the scientific literature addressed only a single hazardous condition (Saegert et al. 2003), despite the fact that many health hazards are co-located in substandard low-income housing. Several reviews show many links between health (both physical and mental) and housing quality, especially with regard to specific chronic diseases and injuries (Breysse et al. 2004; Jacobs 2004; Krieger and Higgins 2002; Matte and Jacobs 2000).

As a result, training, funding, and programs developed over the previous 50 years have been categoric in nature. Strengthening public health infrastructure to make it more effective will depend on aligning policies and strategies that adequately address inefficiencies and limitations. As the public health community increases its emphasis on holistic, prevention-oriented, and population-based approaches, the workforce will require commensurate training. Some key components for training and certification have been developed. In 2006, the CDC and HUD updated the 1975 CDC/American Public Health Association's *Basic Housing Inspection Manual* (US Public Health Service 1975), renaming it the *Healthy Housing Reference Manual* (CDC and HUD 2006). In addition, a "Healthy Homes

Specialist Credential" is now being offered by the National Environmental Health Association (http://www.neha.org/credential/HHS/index.htm) to trainees who successfully complete the Healthy Homes training course offered through the National Healthy Homes Training Center and Network.

THE ROLE OF ENVIRONMENTAL PUBLIC HEALTH PROFESSIONALS

Before World War II, many local health departments had active housing code enforcement programs. These programs were principally related to rental housing units and primarily, if not exclusively, served low-income residents. In many cases, the programs were driven by complaints made by the occupants of the housing units. Health department housing inspectors responding to complaints conducted detailed inspections of the entire dwelling, looking for violations of the department's housing code.

The housing codes of the day were focused on the physical structure. Emphasis was placed on ensuring that the building envelope (roof, walls, foundation, windows, and doors) was properly constructed, capable of bearing the weight of the building, and free of cracks, holes, leaks, or other defects that might permit the entry of the elements or vermin. Inspections identified interior violations, such as problems with sanitation, and exterior violations, including debris and poorly maintained outbuildings. Inspectors also examined the heating, ventilation, plumbing, and electrical systems to ensure they were installed and operating properly. After World War II, there was a dramatic increase in federal funding for new housing, setting off a building boom, particularly of suburban housing developments where there was more land available and lower purchase and development costs. One result of this rush to the suburbs was the neglect and deterioration of many housing units in older, and increasingly perceived as less desirable, parts of the city. These housing units then became the habitation for those too poor to move to the suburbs, people from rural areas, and immigrants and refugees from other countries. With limited resources and little incentive for their occupants or owners to invest in the rental units, these dwellings gradually deteriorated until they were finally deemed unfit for human habitation, in many cases abandoned and the property left vacant or torn down. However, the trend has shifted recently so that more low-income households are in the suburbs (Harvard University 2010).

Local health departments, at least those that continued to have responsibility for enforcing the housing code, were faced with the problem of responding to complaints from renters of property that was often marginal to begin with, owned by absentee landlords or so-called slumlords, that is, individuals or companies that bought dilapidated properties and rented the units to low-income tenants. Because the landlords could always rent out the unit to another tenant, they had little incentive to spend money to make repairs or fix up the unit, and tenants had little incentive to perform routine housekeeping. In response, many cities, such as Pittsburgh, began instituting rent-withholding programs. This allowed a tenant who believed that the landlord was not providing an adequate housing unit to complain to the municipal authority, who would then inspect the housing unit. If sufficient violations of the housing code were found, the landlord would be notified and ordered to make the necessary repairs. Instead of paying rent to the landlord, the tenant's money would go into an escrow account set up by the municipal authority. If the repairs were made in a satisfactory manner by the time allotted by the department, the money would then be paid to the landlord. However, if the repairs were not made, then the money would be returned to the tenant. Rent-withholding programs continue to be used in many municipalities to this day and are one tool to help ensure healthy homes.

However, rent withholding by itself could not solve all of the housing problems. Congress responded to this urban decline with the American Housing Act of 1949 (Title V of P.L. 81–171). Title I of the Act authorized funds to localities to "assist in slum clearance and urban redevelopment" through urban renewal. At their best, urban renewal programs took depressed areas of the inner city and turned them into vibrant, thriving economic communities. At their worst, urban renewal programs demolished broad swaths of urban housing, destroying neighborhoods, churches, schools, community gathering places, and family ties. In the 1970s, Model Cities funding was used by many municipalities to address the problems of a deteriorated housing stock. The Housing and Community Development Act of 1974 created, among other provisions, a new Community Development Block Grant program that consolidated many of the categorically funded HUD programs into a single grant to local governments and states. The Community Development Block Grant programs provided greater flexibility and more local control over the use of HUD funds. However, the funding levels of the combined block grant generally were less than the sum of the previously categorically funded programs.

Many local health departments began divesting themselves of housing code enforcement programs, passing administration and enforcement of the housing code over to separate housing agencies. At the same time, environmental health specialists found that they were being asked to assume new responsibilities in dealing with environmental health issues, many of which were tied to novel funding sources. These included an increase in the number of failing on-site wastewater disposal systems, safeguarding an increasingly complex food supply system and emergency preparedness after the attacks of September 11, 2001. As a result, many health departments got out of the housing business or let it atrophy into a complaint response program relegated to a relatively low priority within the agency.

There has been recent, renewed interest in tackling housing-related problems important to health and well-being (Galster 2008). This renewed interest has come from a number of different directions. Planners, architects, and several citizen groups and nongovernmental organizations now recognize a shared interest in housing and believe that a single-focus approach on one housing problem at a time is inefficient and ineffective. There is a growing appreciation of the need to adopt a holistic approach when dealing with housing issues and to form partnerships with the homeowners and occupants, as well as allied professionals and organizations. Public health agencies, with their expertise in human health and experience in dealing with deteriorating housing stock, play a key role in this effort to preserve, upgrade, and increase affordable housing units.

An example of the type of partnerships that should be developed is the "Master Home Environmentalist Program" of the American Lung Association in Washington (ALAW). This program was originally developed more than 20 years ago through the combined effort of the ALAW, the Young Men's Christian Association, Public Health–Seattle & King County, and the University of Washington's Department of Environmental Health. Together, they adapted the successful Master Home Gardener program concept to train individuals to assess and correct problems in their own homes.

The CDC has provided leadership in the renewed efforts to improve health by improving housing, and together with HUD published the updated and revised *Healthy Housing Reference Manual* (CDC and HUD 2006). The manual provides a brief history of housing, the purpose of housing, and housing regulation. The manual also discusses the American Public Health Association's basic principles of healthy housing before beginning a detailed examination of housing and housing units that provides guidance to the sanitarian and other housing inspectors on the critical aspects of housing structure and its contained housing units and systems.

In 2008, the CDC and HUD jointly published a companion document, the *Healthy Housing Inspection Manual*, which provides a step-by-step guide to inspecting a house. Included in this manual is a sample survey form that can be given to the occupants of a home to gather information on any self-reported health conditions or symptoms that could assist the inspector in identifying potential housing problems. The major portion of the manual consists of a visual assessment data-collection form, which goes through the housing unit, system by system, to identify problems.

The CDC also provided funding that enabled the National Center for Healthy Housing to develop a National Healthy Housing Training Center and Network. The Training Center brought together national experts on housing and health to develop a training program to accomplish its mission. Early in the development, it was agreed that a more holistic approach to looking at housing problems was needed. People from the various organizations and agencies were brought together to build networks and relationships that could help resolve these housing problems through coordinated efforts.

THE ROLE OF HOME VISTING PROFESSIONALS

Florence Nightingale, the founder of modern nursing, was an early proponent of home visiting to improve health outcomes. Nightingale understood that "[t]he connection between the health and the dwelling of the population is one of the most important that exists" and believed that interventions to improve the housing environment would create the conditions within which individuals could become healthy or sustain their health (Lowry 1991). Today, home visiting programs are often staffed by nurses, community health workers, and social workers. In addition, physical therapists and a large number of voluntary programs, such as Meals on Wheels, the Red Cross, and faith-based organizations, provide health and social services in people's homes. Each of these workers is in a unique position to influence the health of the occupants. Although not every program will lend itself to the comprehensive approach described, home visitors are encouraged to identify those assessments and interventions that could be integrated into existing services and to avail themselves of the educational opportunities described later in this chapter.

HOME ASSESSMENT

Home hazards can be assessed in a variety of ways, ranging from self-report to visual inspection to quantitative measurement of specific environmental exposures. Although in many cases home visiting programs may be unable to provide a comprehensive home inspection, existing housing assessment tools could be adapted and linked to the patient assessment tools currently in use. Sample pediatric homes assessment survey forms and nursing care plans can be found at http://www.healthyhomestraining.org/Nurse. Elderly home visiting programs could easily modify these documents for their target population.

Home visitors not only provide home assessment but also serve as a resource for referral and information. First Connections, Rhode Island's Home Visiting Program, is a useful model of incorporating healthy homes services into an existing home visiting program. This risk assessment and referral program identifies children up to three years old who may have poor developmental outcomes. First Connections services are provided by a multidisciplinary team of nurses, social workers, and community health workers. Most families receive 1–4 visits. The team provides home assessments and connection to community services, and helps parents understand and support child development. Approximately one third of the children born in Rhode Island each year are enrolled in the program. One focus of the program is information on detecting and controlling housing-related health and safety hazards. The home visitors also serve as the neighborhood resource for a variety of community-based programs, including the Healthy Housing Program. This home visiting program offers an effective mechanism for parental support. The program also provides a variety of data on the well-being and needs of Rhode Island's young families, data that are crucial to policy development and program evaluation.

WORKFORCE DEVELOPMENT

Although both health and housing programs have recognized the need for an identifiable and trained workforce, at present no sector is charged with developing, implementing, enforcing, and evaluating the introduction of modern healthy homes principles into the housing stock. We explore how existing professional development activities can be adapted to stimulate the birth of a new healthy homes workforce, eliminating a serious policy and capacity gap.

Diffuse responsibility for housing and health across multiple entities that is evident in many communities in most developed countries is further exacerbated by a lack of leadership. This deficiency led the CDC to establish a National Public Health Leadership Development Network (Institute of Medicine 1998, 2003) and to recognize the importance of cross-training and frequent opportunities for collaboration. The major areas of leadership practice and competency identified include the following.

The first area is known as "transorganization," the idea that many public health problems, including inadequate housing, extend beyond the scope of a single stakeholder group, community, profession, organization, or government unit. Thus, health and housing professionals must be effective beyond their immediate fields. For example, within the housing arena, public health professionals are increasingly a voice in urban planning, transportation policy, housing policy and financing, and "green" development. Conversely, within the health field, engineering and building design are increasingly recognized as important interventions that sustain or improve health. In western countries, a "health impact assessment" procedure has been proposed to enable a fuller grasp of the health consequences of community development (Dannenberg et al. 2008). "Transorganization" calls on professionals working in housing and economic development to acquire competency in areas as varied as assessment of radiation hazards and environmental justice.

The second area of competency is "transformation," the ability to identify and implement systematic changes necessary to create the desired outcome through visioning, strategic and tactical alliances, and communication. For example, cross-linking local lists of addresses of lead-poisoned children with lists of addresses of federally subsidized housing is now required under HUD's lead-safe housing regulation (24 CFR Part 35). This system-level change required new alliances to properly balance privacy issues with the need to ensure that public dollars were not inadvertently subsidizing houses that posed health risks.

The third area of competency is legislation and politics. It is noteworthy that, until recently, neither housing nor health has been a leading legislative or political issue in the United States (Wright et al. 2000). The recent mortgage and health insurance crises have led to calls for reform in both arenas, although they still tend to be viewed as separate and disconnected entities, despite the evidence that housing costs compete and often trump health care costs as families, especially low-income ones, struggle with impoverished household budgets. Despite the lack of attention and low priority given to the relationship between health and housing in the policy arena, that relationship was recognized and continued to affect programmatic priorities and initiatives in the United States. The Healthy People 2010 national health goals contain several housing-related objectives, including a call for reducing the 1995 levels of occupied housing units that are substandard by 52% because "residents of substandard housing are at increased risk for fire, electrical injuries, lead poisoning, falls, rat bites, and other illnesses and injuries" (U.S. Department of Health and Human Services 2000). It is expected that similar housing goals will be included in the Healthy People 2020 goals.

Three levels of proficiency in the healthy housing workforce should be established. In general, decision-makers and management staff should achieve an **awareness** level or basic level of mastery of the material. These individuals should be able to identify the concept or skill and understand its importance, although they may have a limited ability to perform the skill. Mid-level supervisors should be knowledgeable, with an intermediate mastery of the material and ability to apply and describe the skill. Front-line workers who actually perform the tasks should be proficient; expected to achieve an expert level of mastery; and able to synthesize, critique, or teach the skill or concept (Table 6.1).

DISCIPLINES IN NEED OF TRAINING

State and local jurisdictions grapple with the intersection of health and housing, and practitioners seeking training and information about healthy homes are challenged because there is no central repository or resource. Moreover, resources directed toward health professionals often neglect the housing component, whereas

TABLE 6.1 — AREAS IN WHICH HEALTHY HOMES PROFESSIONALS SHOULD EXHIBIT A LEVEL OF MASTERY

1. ASSESSMENT SKILLS	4. HAZARD CONTROL MEASURES
• Initial assessment of the home environment using senses (especially smell and sight) • Environmental sampling and measurement in the home • Hazard recognition skills • Resident survey/environmental health history	• Prevention: design, construction, planning, maintenance, renovation • Remediation or intervention • Intervention or actionable hazards • Emergency action items (e.g., carbon monoxide)
2. ANALYTIC SKILLS	5. COMMUNICATION SKILLS/COMMUNITY DIMENSIONS
• Baseline data collection/research on health and environmental factors • Evidence and performance-based outcomes • Program evaluation • Basic computer proficiency	• Active listening skills to actually "hear" the client • Cultural competency skills • Conflict resolution • Training to be a "change" agent • Training and intervention for residents, owners, and community workers • Knowledge of other agencies' roles and responsibilities for collaboration and referrals
3. BACKGROUND KNOWLEDGE	6. ETHICAL, LEGAL, OTHER CONSIDERATIONS
• Basic environmental health • Basic public health • Basic building science • Specific environmental and safety hazards (interior house and exterior built environment) • Specific health effects for children, adults, and elderly	• Personal safety • Ethical and legal considerations • Insurance and liability issues • Code and regulatory issues

TABLE 6.2—PROFESSIONAL DISCIPLINES IN THE UNITED STATES THAT COULD INCORPORATE HEALTHY HOMES PRINCIPLES INTO THEIR EXISTING WORK

Apprentices/trades people	Industrial hygienists
Architects/engineers	Law enforcement
Building code inspectors (new housing construction)	Lead paint risk assessors/inspectors
Child care workers	Physicians
Community-based/public health nurses	Property managers and maintenance staff
Community development corporations	Public health sanitarians
Community organizers	Realtors/insurance/lenders
Community outreach workers	Residential energy conservation specialists
Contractors	Retail housing groups (e.g., Home Depot)
Environment health practitioners	Social workers
Epidemiologists and other researchers	Trade unions
Fire departments	Trade schools (e.g., community colleges, vocational
"Green building" experts	schools)
Housing code inspectors (housing rehabilitation)	Utilities
Home inspectors (private)	Urban planners
Housing rehabilitation designers	Weatherization agencies

information for housing professionals tends to lack the health perspective. This historical disconnect has been ameliorated recently with the development of standardized training curricula (National Center for Healthy Housing 2008). The first step in curriculum development is identification of potential disciplines that could incorporate healthy homes principles into their work and professional development activities (Table 6.2).

ASSESSMENT OF TRAINING NEEDS

Professionals enter homes for a variety of reasons or may refer occupants to professionals from other disciplines, thus creating an opportunity to identify existing conditions that can adversely affect occupants' health status.

A review of available healthy homes training programs was completed before the curriculum development process noted above. A structured survey was disseminated to public health and housing agencies with established training programs to capture information on the course offerings, location, target audiences, training medium, content of the training programs, suitability for modification or adaptation, methods for assessing comprehension of healthy homes concepts and practices, and capacity for distance learning. The survey documented the wide variety of courses available, ranging from 30- to 48-hour, university-based courses to short seminars for child care providers and teachers (National Center for Healthy Housing 2004). The subject matter was equally diverse, including three-day symposia for contractors, consultants, and industrial hygienists on assessment and control of mold and three-hour courses for community health workers, public health nurses, and housing agency staff focused on asthma, injuries, lead poisoning, hazardous materials, and disaster preparedness.

The survey yielded important information related to the development of the training curriculum and training delivery methods. It showed there was no consensus set of healthy homes competencies on which the performance objectives for the training offerings were based. The majority of activities provided specific training on a particular category of healthy housing (e.g., mold or lead) or a broad-based approach focused on awareness of healthy homes topics. The survey did not examine the extent to which training incorporated a formal evaluation, and no published evaluations of the training activities were identified during a literature review of healthy housing–related journal articles.

Developing curricula for a training or educational program can take many forms; there is no perfect model because each model has advantages and disadvantages. Broadly, though, any successful approach will be systematic, objective, and organized, and will likely be based on the following:

1. for whom the program is developed (target audience);
2. what the individual will learn or do (competencies);
3. how the subject content or skills are best learned (infrastructure: methods, activities, resources); and
4. the extent to which the learning has been achieved (evaluation).

CURRICULUM DEVELOPMENT INITIATIVES

Six primary target audiences need to be proficient in key healthy homes principles: environmental health practitioners (e.g., sanitarians, industrial hygienists), public health nurses, housing/code inspectors, and community organizers, along with asset managers and architects/engineers/project managers.

There is considerable variation among the target audiences in terms of their relevant experience and education levels, as well as their communication skills and learning styles (Table 6.3). This suggests that the training materials and delivery method should be designed in a flexible manner and use a variety of teaching methods. A modular approach can ensure that information is at the right level for students. This approach promotes cross-training and collaboration and ensures that the course is designed to appeal to the multidisciplinary needs of the target audience. Problem-solving, case studies, and other types of interactive and "fun" learning are also ways to help make the course material interesting and relevant to students who may be learning the concepts for the first time and to allow participants from various disciplines to interact.

The development of the National Healthy Homes Training Center and Network, supported by the CDC with funding from HUD, promotes nationwide awareness, knowledge, and proficiency in methods to enhance health and safety through improvements to housing. Its mission is to develop and disseminate training that integrates knowledge from the disciplines of health, housing, and the environment. Training is targeted to professionals from the disciplines listed in Table 6.2.

A "learner profile" for each target audience was developed. Learner profiles answer questions about the target audiences' prior education, relevant training and experience, personal and professional characteristics, and logistical information. The learner profiles influence the design and delivery of the training, including, for example, the level of customization that might be necessary, the degree to which audiences could/should be trained together, and the types of materials and delivery methods that the target audiences would find most accessible and acceptable. There are more than a dozen audiences who could benefit from training in healthy homes (Table 6.3).

Other U.S. training activities include the ALAW Healthy House training for builders, renovators, and architects. This training is seven weeks long and addresses dust and moisture issues, ventilation and filtration, and building materials and environmental health. The ALAW also sponsors a volunteer-driven program designed to help people learn more about health risks from pollutants in their home through home assessment. A training curriculum from the Asthma Regional Council of New England provides housing practitioners with information about pests, toxins, moisture, ventilation, and other housing vectors associated with asthma and respiratory disease (Asthma Regional Council of New England 2001). The Center for Environmental Research and Technology at the University of Tulsa developed a one-day course designed for home-based child care providers. It enables child care providers and owner occupants to assess their home environments for potential threats to children's health. This basic training covers moisture control, integrated pest management, environmental tobacco smoke, carbon monoxide, chemical contaminants, and other child safety hazards.

TABLE 6-? PRIMARY TARGET AUDIENCE MATRIX

Target Audience	Relevant Job Responsibilities	Communication Skills	Educational Level	Learning Style	Environmental Health Experience		Housing Experience	Proximity of Audience Members to Each Other
Environmental Health Practitioners (e.g., Sanitarians)	Conduct investigations and respond to complaints involving issues of environmental health and sanitation; prepare cases for referral or conduct immediate enforcement actions; coordinate with other programs; provide information to the public regarding environmental health and sanitation.	Varied	B.S. or higher, varied	Hands-on/interaction	5	3	Varied	Large concentrations in major cities
Housing/Code Inspectors	Ensure safe, structurally sound, and sanitary building construction. Check plans and perform inspections for compliance with codes and laws, as well as county, state, and federal laws.	Varied	H.S.	Hands-on/interaction	2	1	4	Large concentrations in major cities
Community Organizers	Organize activities with neighborhood residents and community-based agencies and conduct educational activities to achieve policy and programmatic change.	High	Varied	Lecture and hands-on	4	2	4	Everywhere
Community-based Nurses	Facilitate, coordinate, and develop systems, processes, and projects that promote health and that respond to community issues and priorities.	High	B.S. or higher, varied	Didactic	3	4	2	Close
Asset Managers	Visit properties to observe their physical condition and the performance of on-site property manager. Assist on-site management in correcting any deficiencies with the project.	Varied	B.S.	Lecture and hands on	2	2	5	Everywhere
Architects/Engineers/Housing Project Manager	Provide technical advice on architecture, building maintenance, material use; participate in annual building inspections; direct and participate in the preparation and implementation of planning, design, construction, and redevelopment projects.	High	B.S. or higher, varied	Lecture and hands-on	3	2	5	Everywhere

*Likert Scale with 5 as the greatest experience and 1 as the least experience.

EVALUATION

No training program is complete without a robust evaluation both in terms of its acceptance by the target audience and whether it has resulted in changes in the participants' professional practice. The overall goal of evaluation is to ensure that public health and housing practitioners receive adequate and appropriate training subjected to continuous improvement.

The following tools can be used to evaluate the training offerings:

- collection of pre- and post-test information about basic healthy housing knowledge of training participants;
- summary of participant feedback on the quality of the educational experience, quality of instruction, appropriateness of tools and curriculum, and satisfaction with the general approach based on a written evaluation tool;
- audit and videotaping of the initial class by project staff; and
- organization of separate unstructured focus groups with students and faculty to ascertain strengths and weaknesses of the training and glean suggested changes for future training.

Student surveys can include metrics for the following:

- satisfaction with the training, including the registration process;
- understanding of core competencies of Healthy Homes professionals;
- the extent to which the curriculum adequately conveyed Healthy Homes theory and practical tools for them to use in their professional positions;
- whether participation in the training created opportunities for networking and expanded collaboration with other professionals on Healthy Homes activities;
- the likelihood that other professionals in their respective organizations (or students in their departments) would participate in further classes;
- perceived barriers to using the content of the coursework;
- preferences for receiving emerging information on Healthy Homes; and
- recommendations for changes to the curriculum.

CONCLUSION

To improve the nation's health, we must improve the nation's housing and ensure the widespread availability of safe, healthy, and affordable housing. A multidisciplinary healthy homes workforce that shares a common set of work practices derived from a science-based framework is essential. Environmental public health, home visiting programs, and housing programs can promote healthy housing by incorporating these practices into their existing protocols and by identifying emerging opportunities to improve those housing factors that affect health.

REFERENCES

Allen, T. Private sector housing improvement in the U.K. and the chronically ill: implications for collaborative working. *Housing Studies* 2005:20(1):63–80.

American Public Health Association Committee on the Hygiene of Housing. *The Basic Principles of Healthful Housing*. 2nd ed. New York, NY: American Public Health Association, Reprinted 1946.

Asthma Regional Council of New England. *Healthy and Affordable Housing Training Practical Recommendations for Building, Renovating and Maintaining Housing*. Boston, MA: Asthma Regional Council, 2001. Available at: http://www.asthmaregionalcouncil.org/about/housingtraining.html. Accessed November 29, 2004.

Breysse, P., L. Bergofsky, W. Galke, N. Farr, and R. Morley. The relationship between housing and health: Children at risk. *Environ Health Perspect* 2004:112(15):1583.

Centers for Disease Control and Prevention and U.S. Department of Housing and Urban Development. *Healthy Housing Inspection Manual*. Atlanta, GA: U.S. Department of Health and Human Services, 2008.

——. *Healthy Housing Reference Manual*. Atlanta, GA: U.S. Department of Health and Human Services, 2006. Available at: http://www.cdc.gov/nceh/publications/books/housing/housing.htm. Accessed March 29, 2008.

Dannenberg, A.L., R. Bhatia, B.L. Cole, S.K. Heaton, J.D. Feldman, and C.D. Rutt. Use of health impact assessment in the U.S.: 27 case studies, 1999–2007. *Am J Prev Med* 2008:34(3):241–56.

Galster, G.C. U.S. housing scholarship, planning and policy since 1968. *J Am Plann Assoc* 2008:74(1):5–16.

Harvard University Joint Center for Housing Studies. State of the Nation's Housing, 2010. Cambridge, MA. 2010. Available at: http://www.jchs.harvard.edu/son/index.htm. Accessed June 18, 2010.

Institute of Medicine. *The Future of Public Health. Committee for the Study of the Future of Public Health*. Washington, DC: National Academy Press, 1998.

——. *Who Will Keep the Public Healthy? Educating Public Health Professionals for the 21st Century*. Washington, DC: National Academy Press, 2003.

Jacobs, D.E. *Housing and Health: Challenges and Opportunities*. Proceedings of the World Health Organization Symposium on Housing and Health, October 1, 2004, Vilnius, Lithuania.

Krieger, J., and D. Higgins. Housing and health: Time again for public health action. *Am J Public Health* 2002:92:5.

LookLex Encyclopedia. *Code of Hammurabi, c. 1780 B.C.E* (June 2009). Available at: http://looklex.com/e.o/hammurabi.htm.

Lowry, S. Housing. *BMJ* 1991:303(6806):838–40.

Matte, T.D., and D.E. Jacobs. Housing and health—current issues and implications for research and programs. *J Urban Health* 2000:77(1):7–25.

National Center for Healthy Housing. *Blueprint for Success: Work Group Report of the Healthy Homes Training Center and Network.* Columbia, MD: National Center for Healthy Housing, 2004. Available at: http://www.nchh.org/LinkClick.aspx?fileticket=rs1iUR2e%2F%2FA%3D&tabid=298. Accessed August 6, 2010.

———. Fact Sheet: National Healthy Homes Training Center and Network. (2010). Available at: http://www.healthyhomestraining.org/Practitioner/HHTC_Brochure_2-10.pdf. Accessed August 5, 2010.

Saegert, S.C., S. Klitzman, N. Freudenberg, J. Cooperman-Mroczek, and S. Nasser. Healthy housing: A structured review of published evaluations of US interventions to improve health by modifying housing in the United States, 1990–2001. *Am J Public Health* 2003:93:1471–7.

U.S. Department of Health and Human Services, Office of Disease Prevention and Health Promotion. *Healthy People 2010 Objectives for the Nation.* Atlanta, GA: U.S. Department of Health and Human Services, Office of Disease Prevention and Health Promotion, 2000. Available at: http://www.health.gov/healthypeople/. Accessed November 24, 2004.

U.S. Public Health Service. APHA-CDC recommended housing maintenance and occupancy ordinance. Atlanta: US Department of Health and Human Services; 1975.

Wright, K., L. Rowitz, A. Merkle, et al. Competency development in public health leadership. *Am J Public Health* 2000:90:1202–7.

Cooperative Extension Agencies and Community Health Education

Joseph Wysocki, PhD, and Joseph Ponessa, PhD

The Cooperative Extension System (CES) of the U.S. Department of Agriculture (USDA) was established by Congress through the enactment of the Smith-Lever Act and signed into law by President Woodrow Wilson on May 8, 1914. In the past century, the CES has evolved into the only comprehensive national infrastructure in the world that links individual citizens and communities with their public universities and all levels of government in a mutual and continuous applied learning relationship. As its name indicates, there are two critical factors that are key to the CES and its success: cooperation and extension.

The CES is a *cooperative* educational partnership among all levels of government, including the United States federal partner, the USDA Cooperative State Research, Education, and Extension Service (CSREES), which on October 1, 2009, became the National Institute for Food and Agriculture; the state governments through the land-grant universities; and county and local governments. The CES has offices in more than 2,900 of our nation's counties.

The CES is an *extension* because as an organization it is designed to extend or reach out with knowledge from the land-grant university to the people of the state. The information offered by Extension is provided by scientists and researchers at the university and is made practical and relevant by Extension educators or agents who are located in each county Extension office and are in direct contact with their clients and stakeholders.

The CES is built on a cadre of subject matter specialists, based in land-grant universities, historically African American universities, and tribal institutions in every U.S. state and territory. The information that the CES develops, on the basis of national priorities and local, client-based inputs, is disseminated to general and specific audiences, both lay and professional, through a system of county-based outreach agents in most counties throughout the country. The established client base views this system as a source of accurate and unbiased information, and the CES is generally viewed as a trusted resource. Specialists and agents are also constantly seeking new audiences and modalities to disseminate current, practical information.

LAND-GRANT UNIVERSITIES

Land-grant universities are institutions of higher education that have been designated by each state to receive the benefits of the Morrill Acts of 1862 and 1890 (Rasmussen 1989). These acts supported the development of institutions of higher education in all states by granting them federally controlled land that could then be used to fund the institutions. The land-grant universities are fundamental to the organizational structure and success of the CES, because the educational base of practical knowledge and information resulting from scholarship and research at these universities is extended into the community through outreach efforts of the county educators or agents.

Land-grant institutions are often categorized as 1862, 1890, or 1994, according to the year of the legislation that established their land-grant status. Today, this list includes the following 108 institutions.

1862: There are 57 land grants, one for each state, the District of Columbia, plus the territories.

1890: These are the 18 historically African American universities.

1994: The most recent land grants are the 33 Native American institutions.

A complete listing of the land grants is included in Table 7.1.

There are approximately 4,000 state Extension specialists and 9,000 county Extension educators (personal communication, Dr. James C. Wade, Director, Extension and Outreach, Association of Public and Land-Grant Universities). In addition, the federal partner of the Extension system has a staff of fewer than 400 people in Washington, DC, who have program responsibilities related to research and higher education in addition to Extension responsibilities. An integral part of the Morrill Act is the Hatch Act of 1887, which created the Agricultural Experiment Stations. The Experiment Stations have been a foundation of research for the CES.

TABLE 7.1—LAND-GRANT COLLEGES AND UNIVERSITIES (1862, 1890, AND 1994)

Alabama
Alabama A&M University, Normal
Auburn University, Auburn
Tuskegee University, Tuskegee

Alaska
Ilisagvik College, Barrow
University of Alaska, Fairbanks

American Samoa
American Samoa Community
College, Pago Pago

Arizona
Diné College, Tsaile
University of Arizona, Tucson
Tohono O'Odham Community
College, Sells

Arkansas
University of Arkansas, Fayetteville
University of Arkansas, Pine
Bluff

California
D-Q University, (Davis vicinity)
University of California System-
Oakland as Headquarters, Oakland

Colorado
Colorado State University, Fort
Collins

Connecticut
University of Connecticut, Storrs

Delaware
Delaware State University, Dover
University of Delaware, Newark

District of Columbia
University of the District of
Columbia, Washington

Florida
Florida A&M University, Tallahassee
University of Florida, Gainesville

Georgia
Fort Valley State University, Fort
Valley
University of Georgia, Athens

Guam
University of Guam, Mangilao

Hawaii
University of Hawaii, Honolulu

Idaho
University of Idaho, Moscow

Illinois
University of Illinois, Urbana

Indiana
Purdue University, West Lafayette

Iowa
Iowa State University, Ames

Kansas
Haskell Indian Nations University,
Lawrence
Kansas State University, Manhattan

Kentucky
Kentucky State University,
Frankfort
University of Kentucky, Lexington

Louisiana
Louisiana State University, Baton
Rouge
Southern University and A&M
College, Baton Rouge

Maine
University of Maine, Orono

Maryland
University of Maryland, College
Park
University of Maryland Eastern
Shore, Princess Anne

Massachusetts
University of Massachusetts,
Amherst

Michigan
Bay Mills Community College,
Brimely
Michigan State University, East
Lansing
Saginaw Chippewa Tribal College,
Mount Pleasant

Micronesia
College of Micronesia, Kolonia,
Pohnpei

Minnesota
Fond du Lac Tribal & Community
College, Cloquet
Leech Lake Tribal College, Cass
Lake
University of Minnesota, St. Paul
White Earth Tribal and Community
College, Mahnomen

TABLE 7.1 — (CONTINUED)

Mississippi
Alcorn State University, Lorman
Mississippi State University,
Mississippi State

Missouri
Lincoln University, Jefferson City
University of Missouri, Columbia

Montana
Blackfeet Community College,
Browning
Chief Dull Knife College, Lame Deer
Fort Belknap College, Harlem
Fort Peck Community College, Poplar
Little Big Horn College, Crow Agency
Montana State University, Bozeman
Salish Kootenai College, Pablo
Stone Child College, Box Elder

Nebraska
Little Priest Tribal College,
Winnebago
Nebraska Indian Community
College, Winnebago
University of Nebraska, Lincoln

Nevada
University of Nevada, Reno

New Hampshire
University of New Hampshire,
Durham

New Jersey
Rutgers University, New Brunswick

New Mexico
Navajo Technical College, Crownpoint

Institute of American Indian Arts,
Sante Fe
New Mexico State University,
Las Cruces
Southwestern Indian Polytechnic
Institute, Albuquerque

New York
Cornell University, Ithaca

North Carolina
North Carolina A&T State
University, Greensboro
North Carolina State University,
Raleigh

North Dakota
Fort Berthold Community College,
New Town
Cankdeska Cikana Community
College, Fort Totten
North Dakota State University,
Fargo
Sitting Bull College, Fort Yates
Turtle Mountain Community
College, Belcourt
United Tribes Technical College,
Bismarck

Northern Marianas
Northern Marianas College, Saipan,
CM

Ohio
Ohio State University, Columbus

Oklahoma
Langston University, Langston
Oklahoma State University,
Stillwater

Oregon
Oregon State University, Corvallis

Pennsylvania
Pennsylvania State University,
University Park

Puerto Rico
University of Puerto Rico, Mayaguez

Rhode Island
University of Rhode Island, Kingston

South Carolina
Clemson University, Clemson
South Carolina State University,
Orangeburg

South Dakota
Oglala Lakota College, Kyle
Si Tanka University, Eagle Butte
Sinte Gleska University, Rosebud
Sisseton Wahpeton Community
College, Sisseton
South Dakota State University,
Brookings

Tennessee
Tennessee State University,
Nashville
University of Tennessee, Knoxville

Texas
Prairie View A&M University, Prairie
View
Texas A&M University, College Station

Utah
Utah State University, Logan

TABLE 7.1 — (CONTINUED)

Vermont	**Washington**	**Wisconsin**
University of Vermont, Burlington	Northwest Indian College, Bellingham	College of Menominee Nation, Keshena
Virgin Islands	Washington State University, Pullman	Lac Courte Oreilles Ojibwa, Community College, Hayward
University of the Virgin Islands, St. Croix		University of Wisconsin, Madison
	West Virginia	
Virginia	West Virginia State University, Institute	**Wyoming**
Virginia Polytechnic Institute and State University, Blacksburg	West Virginia University, Morgantown	University of Wyoming Laramie, WY
Virginia State University, Petersburg		

Source: *U.S. Department of Agriculture, Cooperative State Research, Education, and Extension Service.*

FUNDING FOR THE COOPERATIVE EXTENSION SYSTEM

The funding for the CES comes from three primary sources. Both the land-grant universities and the local county Extension offices are supported by the USDA CSREES, which distributes annually congressionally appropriated formula grants to supplement state and county funds. CSREES affects how these formula grants are used through national program leadership to help identify timely national priorities and ways to address these issues. In this cooperative partnership, state funds are used to support the state land-grant universities (with some states having more than one land-grant university), and county funds are also provided to support programs at the local level. In recent years, the percentage of federal and state funds has become a smaller portion of the support for many state Extension services; Extension services in those states have had to find other resources and ways to supplement their programs, including grants, awards, and contracts with other agencies and entities. In some cases, state Extension services have begun charging fees for services and materials.

CONSTITUENCIES SERVED BY THE COOPERATIVE EXTENSION SYSTEM

In addition to serving the public at large, the CES serves a wide variety of constituencies and audiences. Extension agents and subject matter specialists will often seek out special audiences and collaborative partners as part of their mandate to convey useful information to the public. Special audiences include, for example, nonprofit groups and nongovernment organizations, schools (public and private), and state and local (as well as federal) government entities at every level. Assistance can also be rendered to businesses (with certain limitations) and professional groups.

In the organizational structure of the CES, expertise in matters involving healthy housing will nearly always fall within the purview of the housing specialist, although not all housing specialists count healthy housing issues among their responsibilities. In some instances, a county agent with special interest or training in this area will take on such responsibilities and may assume a regional or statewide outreach role.

Although Extension programs and offices are located in urban and suburban communities, it is in rural areas and at the local and county levels that Extension educational programs make their most innovative contributions. No other federal agency has the educational outreach and service delivery systems, as well as partnership with the land-grant university, that are found with the Extension service. Furthermore, there are several housing issues in the rural community that the Extension service is unique in addressing. In the mid-1990s, USDA's CSREES partnered with USDA's Natural Resource Conservation Service and the U.S. Environmental Protection Agency (EPA) to develop a national program on rural housing environmental and health-related issues that was implemented at the local level in rural communities by the Extension service. The program "Home*A*Syst" educated the public about the following issues: site assessment and protection of water quality around a home; storm-water management, including reducing pollutants in runoff; drinking well-water management, including well location, construction, maintenance, testing, and unused wells; household wastewater management, including septic systems design, location, and maintenance; liquid fuels management; indoor environmental quality and health; and fertilizer and pesticide use and storage.Because mobile and manufactured homes are often located in rural communities, the Extension service also addresses the health-related issues with this type of housing.

Rendered services can be in the form of informational meetings, publications, or specific problem-solving advice. Staff trainings are another modality of outreach, often rendered to professional associations, community health groups, and community outreach workers (in a train-the-trainer format). Relationships are often established with state and local health departments; assistance can range from technical help with public queries to training of health department staff and related professionals, such as school nurses. Health department collaborations are sometimes established in times of emergency, such as flooding/post-flood cleanup, when there is an immediate public need for trusted, authoritative information.

Advice and assistance are also given to small businesses, within reasonable limits, making sure that no prejudice or favoritism is shown.

Other forms that Extension outreach and assistance can take include curriculum development and sharing, as well as expert review of manuscripts and curricula. Fact sheets, brochures, and various electronic media are other venues for fulfilling the Extension mandate to disseminate information that is valuable, timely, and research based.

According to the context of this mandate, information is provided in an objective format (pros and cons, as appropriate) so that the recipients of the information are better equipped to make their own decisions on applications and use. Advocacy positions are to be avoided in CES outreach.

PARTNERSHIPS TO ADVANCE HEALTHY AND SAFE HOUSING

Integral to the CES is the concept of partnerships and connecting with others who share common missions to produce the desired educational results. The CES partners include other federal agencies, private organizations, and state and local agencies. Some examples of national and international programs illustrate the scope and diversity of Extension activity in the area of healthy housing.

Radon Programs

Extension responses ranged from conducting public awareness seminars to training radon professionals to establishing EPA radon training centers around the country. Many states received EPA funding to conduct these programs, and efforts continue to this day. In some states, the CES is designated as the lead agency dealing with this issue; in others, there is close collaboration with the state radon agency or state health department.

National Healthy Homes Training Center

Approximately six state land-grant institutions participate in the National Healthy Homes Training Center of the National Center for Healthy Housing http://www.nchh.org). These collaborating universities assist with multi-day training sessions for health and housing professionals, providing conference management and instructional support for these regional training sessions. Trainees conduct educational classes and other outreach in their communities. Credentialing for participants is also available through a partnership between the National Center for Healthy Housing and the National Environmental Health Association.

Demonstration Houses

There have been two major developments in residential structures over the last several decades: (1) recognition that the indoor environment can pose serious hazards to human health and (2) major advances in building science (showing research-based "best practices" for economically constructing safe, healthy, and sustainable dwellings). Promulgating these concepts among homebuilders and those seeking housing takes many forms. One approach is to develop "demonstration houses" that incorporate these principles and are used as community educational resources. In collaboration with a wide array of partners, the CES has developed such homes in several states, usually under the aegis of the state university. Such projects include the following:

- Utah House (http://www.theutahhouse.org): A planning project was initiated by Utah State University Extension in 1996, when a planning team of 50 volunteers formed committees to work on marketing, education, fundraising, infrastructure, house design, and landscape design. A design team was assembled to develop overall concepts for the project, and a major fund-raising effort was launched. Ground was broken in 2001, and the building was completed in 2003. Educational outreach is provided to youth and adult audiences, covering topics ranging from energy conservation and geothermal basics to sustainable living and the indoor environment. This facility is situated in the Utah Botanical Center, and there is primary emphasis on outdoor ecological issues. To date, 10,000 visitors have come through this facility.

- LaHouse (http://www.lsuagcenter.com/en/family_home/home/la_house): The LaHouse began with a contingent of Louisiana State University Agricultural Center experts from within and outside of Extension. Disciplines included housing and engineering, environmental sciences, disaster mitigation, entomology, and educational outreach. Other researchers were brought in as well, along with key state and federal representatives and funding partners. The goals of the project are to demonstrate practical ways to attain comfort, durability, value, convenience, and better health, while reducing the use of water and energy, pollution, waste, and property damage. The healthy aspects include both indoor environmental quality and universal design. A wide range of educational resources are provided to youth, adults, and professionals.

- Florida House (http://www.Sarasota.extension.uf.edu/FHLC/FlaHouseHome.shtml): This is a similar project involving hundreds of organizations, government agencies, businesses, and individuals. Originally inspired by the need for a better way to promote water conservation, Florida House has evolved into a broad demonstration of sustainability principles, including durability (against hurricanes and insect infestations), energy conservation, and the selection of least toxic building materials and furnishings. Indoor environmental quality is an important component of its educational outreach.

Healthy Homes Partnership

The Healthy Homes Partnership is a public outreach education program that links the resources of the USDA/CSREES and state land-grant universities with the U.S. Department of Housing and Urban Development (HUD), Office of Healthy Homes and Lead Hazard Control, as part of HUD's Healthy Homes Program Initiative. The goal of this project is to promote the health and safety of children in the home environment through educational outreach. The project is funded through a cooperative agreement between CSREES and HUD; in the 10 years of its existence it has relayed approximately $2.8 million to project managers in 30 states and the Virgin Islands. Local outreach educational efforts have involved partnerships with numerous local agencies and partners at the national, state, and community/county levels. One of the major products of this initiative is the booklet "Help Yourself to a Healthy Home" (http://www.healthyhomespartnership.net/book.html). This publication, aimed at low-literacy audiences, is now in its third edition and available in six languages, with a special edition aimed at Native American audiences. The booklet is targeted to parents and caregivers, and addresses several high-impact issues affecting children's health. It is a mainstay of the Healthy Homes project and is also in use by health departments, community-based organizations across the nation, and several foreign countries (personal communication, L. Booth, Healthy Homes Partnership National Coordinator, Alabama Cooperative Extension System, Auburn University, Alabama).

Healthy Indoor Air for America's Homes

The Healthy Indoor Air for America's Homes project, a public education initiative that began in 1996, is the result of a cooperative agreement between the USDA–CSREES and the EPA (http://www.csrees.udsa.gov/nea/family/in_focus/housing_if_epa/html). The initiative's core purpose was to provide the nationwide, county-based system of Extension educators with the means to address a mutually expressed need (along with the EPA) to disseminate information on indoor environmental quality. A team of six Extension housing specialists from around the country, along with the project leader, spent a year preparing training materials, including curricula, promotional and evaluation material, related fact sheets, and a set of Frequently Asked Questions posed to the site over the years (http://www.healthyindoorair.org). An initial training was provided to Extension state program leaders and other stakeholders from each state, who then provided training and support materials to county agents and others for presentation to the public on a variety of indoor environmental topics. In the ensuing 2 years, the original participants trained an additional 2,500 Extension educators and reached more than 15,000 professionals. In the decade that this program existed, train-the-trainer sessions have been provided to 169,714 individuals. Professionals trained include more than 12,000 health department officials, 13,000 teachers, 12,202 real estate professionals, 12,809 builders, and 104,230 others, including child care providers and staff members of organizations, such as the American Lung Association. Many of these trainings evolved into ongoing collaborative relationships with these groups. Although it has proved impossible to tabulate all of the collaborating groups and entities that partnered with the CES in this project, the 10-year accomplishment report lists more than 40 groups and categories of groups (e.g., Habitat for Humanity, hospitals, construction firms, and utilities) that have assisted in various ways (U.S. EPA 2006).

Other Resources

The CES has identified flooding and other disasters affecting substantial numbers of citizens in different parts of the country at different times as a major outreach initiative. As a result, comprehensive packages of information (usually rendered as organized collections of short, readily accessible fact sheets) on a variety of disaster types have been available for some time. This body of information is collected under the aegis of the Extension Disaster Education Network (EDEN) and is now available online. The flooding module, which addresses health issues in the context of the short- and long-term flood recovery process, is available from the EDEN gateway (http://www.eden.lsu.edu/default.aspx).

Perhaps Extension's most ambitious electronic outreach involves a much broader information resource being developed under the Wikipedia format. In this venture, known as "eXtension," teams of Extension experts from across the nation are developing comprehensive resources in a wide range of topics. This project is in a relatively early stage of development; a flooding module complements the EDEN information (http://www.extension.org/disasters; this page will open in a page from the land-grant university of the state from which the computer request originates, making it easier to access local information from that institution). A new unit on home energy recently launched, and it is expected that additional Healthy Housing topics will be posted in the future.

ACCESSING EXTENSION OFFICES

The easiest and perhaps the most direct way to locate a county or state Extension office is to visit the federal partner website (http://www.csrees.usda.gov). Go to Quick Links and click on Local Extension Offices or State Partners (http://www.csrees.usda.gov/qlinks/partners/state_partners.html).

Partnerships with Extension personnel may involve subject-matter (e.g., housing) specialists, who are typically located at the state colleges/universities, or agents, who are usually based in counties. Many states, but not all, have initiatives and outreach programs dealing with healthy homes. In some states, these programs are conducted by the specialist; in many instances, however, there is also statewide involvement of county agents.

Although the traditional form of outreach is common, a wide variety of other modalities have been implemented. These include video presentations, distance learning, and other approaches described in the preceding section. Many of these outreach efforts, particularly the larger ones, are grant funded.

There are a number of ways to identify and contact CES personnel. In the realm of health, much of Extension's activities center around issues of food and nutrition, with special interest on low-income food and nutrition issues and physical activity and exercise. In the area of healthy housing, this work may be based in the university with Family and Consumer Sciences or in Engineering units. County CES offices are listed in the "Government" section of the phone directory ("blue pages") in the County Government listings. In some locations, offices may be listed in the white pages under a particular state university. For information on ongoing programs, click on the "Family, Youth & Communities" link on the CSREES website (http://www.csrees.usda.gov). Another link to explore is "Pest Management" for integrated pest management information. Although most efforts in this topic involve agricultural audiences, some states have initiatives on urban integrated pest management. The CSREES site contains a wealth of information on the scope of Extension programs, as well as details of successful programs and partnerships and information on funding opportunities.

Extension personnel are enthusiastic about establishing partnerships and collaborations. These are seen as a good means of fulfilling the Extension mandate to disseminate information. It is useful for potential partners to know about some of the important elements that make such partnerships attractive to Extension. The most important need for Extension is to be able to show beneficial impacts resulting from an outreach effort. Impact indicators include money saved, health improved (e.g., fewer asthma visits to the emergency department), public health improved (e.g., radon tests conducted), and health outreach workers trained (and the multiplier of total audiences reached by the trainees). Thus, the extent to which a partner can facilitate or enhance documented impacts of the project comprises an important benefit to Extension. Partnerships that bring new audiences to Extension are also beneficial (not to mention new funding sources). Likewise, partnerships that bring information or other capabilities that move the project forward are also sought. Such collaborations are mutually beneficial, and credit and acknowledgement are readily given.

As part of Extension's outreach responsibility, pro bono professional training is often provided to personnel of agencies, nonprofit organizations, and other entities; however, follow-up information regarding the implementation and outcomes of such training is often required. Although Extension personnel are usually inclined toward collaborations, there may be instances when collaboration is not possible. With regard to healthy homes–related projects, some housing specialists (or county agents) may not have the background or interest in this area. Others may be constrained by organizational limitations (e.g., previous commitments) or the need for adherence to plans of work in other areas. Another limiting factor is funding; in some states, grant-funded projects may be given preference over those that are not funded. Partnerships involving commercial entities may also be problematic. Although such partnerships can take place, Extension, as a federally sponsored entity, cannot be involved in a program that endorses or otherwise supports an individual company or commercial product. (Likewise, Extension involvement would be inappropriate in a situation in which direct support would be provided to one side of a political controversy or candidate, instead of simply providing objective, fact-based information.) Even when one or more of these constraints are in effect, the Extension professional may be able to provide leads to other potential collaborators.

CONCLUSION

The CES concept is unique in education in that it links citizens and communities with their public universities and three levels of government (federal, state, and local) in an applied learning relationship. An integral part of CES are the 108 land-grant universities located in every U.S. state and the territories. Financing is provided by all three levels of government, supplemented by grants, awards, and contracts. Extension subject matter specialists at these universities work closely with a network of county-based Extension educators who have a long-term, trusting relationship with community residents. With input from national and state partners, local stakeholders, who are representative of the local population, help decide which local programs are needed. This unique relationship is the basis for a time-tested, effective outreach that brings practical university research on current problems to statewide audiences.

During the last two decades, the Extension system has undertaken an increased role in the area of indoor environmental quality and healthy housing issues. Significant accomplishments have been attained, often through collaboration with other entities. Given CES's core mission of conveying research-based, objective information to the public (as well as to professional audiences), partnerships and collaborations that can enhance this outreach are always welcome. Other entities that share the goals and objectives of CES are encouraged to make contact with Extension and explore areas of mutual benefit.

REFERENCES

Rasmussen, W.D. *Taking the University to the People*. Ames, IA: Iowa State University Press, 1989.

U.S. Environmental Protection Agency. *Ten Years of Accomplishments 1995–2005. Final Report, Healthy Indoor Air for America's Homes*. U.S. Environmental Protection Agency, Bozeman, MT: Montana State University USDA-CSREES, 2006.

Green Building and the Code

Lynn Underwood, BA, BS, and Daniel Morrison, BS

The history of housing regulation has been briefly described in previous work (Centers for Disease Control and Prevention and U.S. Department of Housing and Urban Development 2006). As that work noted, the first known housing laws were established in Babylon circa 1792–1750 B.C. The laws addressed the responsibility of the home builder to construct a quality home. In general, building codes were first devised as a way to ensure some acceptable minimum level of safety and sanitation. Plumbing, electrical, and general housing codes ensure health and safety while also minimizing damage to buildings under catastrophic natural disasters, such as floods and earthquakes. Sanitation codes historically have been used to improve health conditions, particularly in large cities. New developments in codes try to go beyond basic health and safety. Energy codes, introduced in the 1970s, were a step toward integrating conservation concerns into codes. Green building codes try to minimize the harm to the environment in the process of home building and to create homes that take as little as possible from the environment. The most important part of the housing code, however, is dictating minimums while maintaining housing affordability.

Building codes have been historically regulated at the local or state level in all 50 states. Three separate major codes developed by different associations arose in the early twentieth century—the Uniform Building Code, the Southern Building Code Conference International, and the Building Officials and Code Administrators International Inc., National Building Code. In addition, in 1952, the American Public Health Association (APHA) Committee on the Hygiene of Housing published a proposed housing ordinance. The ordinance provided a prototype on which legislation might be based and has served as the basis for countless housing codes enacted in the United States since that time. The APHA ordinance was revised over time, and the most recent model ordinance was published by the APHA in 1986 as *Housing and Health: APHA-CDC Recommended Minimum Housing Standards*. It was one of several model ordinances available to communities interested in adopting a housing code (Mood 1986).

A growing need for more consistency across localities led to model codes that crossed large regions of the country. The Conference of American Building Officials, a consortium of Building Officials and Code Administrators International Inc., Southern Building Code Conference International, and International Conference of Building Officials, developed a model code for one- and two-family dwellings in 1983. Although the code was an improvement, builders, architects, and engineers remained challenged by different state codes. Worse, the different state codes meant that various parts of the United States had higher or lower standards for safety, sanitation, and health. The situation improved dramatically, however, with the advent of the International Code Council's International Residential Code (IRC) in 2000. The IRC is a stand-alone codebook that is the reference document for new one- and two-family homes. The IRC includes architectural, structural, energy-efficiency, plumbing, mechanical, gas, and electrical provisions all in one book, but for new construction. The IRC is the main reference document for the production home builder. Although the IRC is dedicated to safety, it weighs in on health and sanitation in a variety of ways. For example, the IRC establishes light, ventilation, and heating standards as well as minimum sanitation rules, including toilet room and kitchen requirements (Table 8.1). The IRC, now in its 4th edition, has been adopted statewide in 37 states and the District of Columbia, as well as localities of 11 additional states. The country is more consistent in building code enforcement than ever before. Although a model code helps establish uniformity across the continent, each jurisdiction tends to amend the code to reflect local tradition, custom, or circumstances. Because of this, building codes still sometimes conflict across city, county, or state boundaries. Over time, these boundary disputes will decrease, but they will always be present in some form. Because of state autonomy guaranteed by the Constitution, it is unlikely there will be a federally enforced building code across all 50 states. Building officials across the country should continue to work toward consistency as more states decrease local amendments.

The International Property Maintenance Code (IPMC), first published by the International Code Council in 1988, establishes minimum standards for all buildings to protect resident health, safety, and welfare, although in practice the code emphasizes safety over health and welfare. The IPMC covers a wide range of property conditions, such as noxious weeds, proper drainage, rodent harborage, exhaust fans, sanitation, roof drainage, window and door condition, insect screens

TABLE 8.1—INTERNATIONAL RESIDENTIAL CODE PROVISION EXAMPLES

Area	Provision
Ventilation	Ventilation of habitable rooms. This can be accomplished with operable windows or mechanical ventilation. Separation of attached garages from living space reduces the risk of vehicle exhaust entering the home. Carbon monoxide detectors are required in some situations. Range hoods are now required for kitchen cooking equipment.
Moisture	Foam plastic with volatile organic compounds is regulated with a thermal barrier or appropriate use. Capillary breaks between foundations and mudsills slow water movement. Pressure-treated mudsills protect against structural decay. Termite management in appropriate areas also protects a structure. Flood-resistant construction standards mitigate damage caused by most non-severe floods. Building science principles have led to alternate weather protection barriers that keep exterior walls dry.
Energy Conservation	A new requirement establishes a blower door test to ensure the tightness of the construction, thus decreasing infiltration of particulate matter from the atmosphere. In addition, ducts in unconditioned attics or crawl spaces are now required to be tested for tightness. Combustion air requirements that normally are satisfied by outdoor air can use certain indoor air, thus reducing penetrations in the environmental envelope. Exhaust ducts are required for gas-producing equipment and clothes dryers, again, to improve the indoor air quality.
Sanitation and Water Quality	Water quality is regulated by preventing cross-connections. Unsanitary conditions caused by sewerage are controlled in a variety of ways, including proper drain, waste, and vent pipe materials and installation. Water heaters must have a pan for water leaks.
Mitigation and Control of Radon	Radon control is required in areas designated by the local jurisdiction. Soil gas retarder (e.g., a polyethylene sheet) lessens infiltration. Vent pipe is specified to carry away harmful gas. Floor openings (e.g., bathtubs, showers, and water closets) are sealed to retard gas entry into the habitable rooms.

in habitable rooms, and food preparation areas (see examples in Table 8.2). The IPMC requires that exterior flaking or peeling paint be corrected to maintain the weather protection barrier and avoid water damage. This provision is also used to encourage property owners to properly maintain lead-based paint in homes built before 1978. The IPMC also regulates light, sanitation, space heating, ventilation, and overcrowding, similar to the IRC.

TABLE 8.2—RELEVANT INTERNATIONAL PROPERTY MAINTENANCE CODE HEALTHY HOME REQUIREMENT EXAMPLES

Area	Provision
Extermination	The control and elimination of insects, rats, or other pests by eliminating their harborage places; by removing or making inaccessible materials that serve as their food; by poison spraying, fumigating, trapping, or any other approved pest elimination methods.
Infestation	The presence, within or contiguous to a structure or premises, of insects, rats, vermin, or other pests.
Sanitation	All exterior property and premises shall be maintained in a clean, safe, and sanitary condition. The occupant shall keep that part of the exterior property that such occupant occupies or controls in a clean and sanitary condition.
Grading and Drainage	All premises shall be graded and maintained to prevent the erosion of soil and the accumulation of stagnant water thereon or within any structure located thereon.
Roofs and Drainage	The roof and flashing shall be sound and tight and not have defects that admit rain. Roof drainage shall be adequate to prevent dampness or deterioration in the walls or interior portion of the structure. Roof drains, gutters, and downspouts shall be maintained in good repair and free from obstructions. Roofwater shall not be discharged in a manner that creates a public nuisance.
Interior Surfaces	All interior surfaces, including windows and doors, shall be maintained in good, clean, and sanitary condition. Peeling, chipping, flaking, or abraded paint shall be repaired, removed, or covered. Cracked or loose plaster, decayed wood, and other defective surface conditions shall be corrected.
Habitable Spaces	Every habitable space shall have at least one openable window. The total openable area of the window in every room shall be equal to at least 45% of the minimum glazed area required in section 402.1.
Energy Conservation Devices	Devices intended to reduce fuel consumption by attachment to a fuel-burning appliance, to the fuel supply line thereto, or to the vent outlet or vent piping therefrom shall not be installed unless labeled for such purpose and the installation is specifically approved.

Source: International Code Council's International Property Maintenance Standards
(http://www.healthyhomestraining.org/Codes/IPMC.htm).

Sanitation codes are generally enacted by a city or state government. The goal of these codes is similar to those established in the Property Maintenance Code, that is, to maintain basic cleanliness in the areas where we live, work, dine, or play. The distinction between a sanitation code and a building code is the focus of the code itself, as well as the responsibility for enforcement. A sanitation code targets the activity that should promote cleanliness, such as the practices of employees at a restaurant: Did the employee wash his or her hands? Is the food preparation area cleaned at proper intervals? Is the floor mopped at specific times? A building code or property maintenance code, however, would ensure that the proper equipment or appliance was installed to make these sanitation efforts possible. For example, is the grease trap installed in a restaurant likely to accumulate fats and greases? Is a hand sink installed in the kitchen of a restaurant? Are the walls in a bathroom smooth, hard, and nonabsorbent so they can be easily washed? These codes work together but have different approaches. In addition, different authorities enforce the codes (e.g., the sanitation code is under the Health Department purview).

HOUSING CODES AND THE ENERGY CRISIS OF THE 1970S

Energy conservation did not make it into the code until energy became scarce. The energy crisis in the United States between 1973 and 1974 had a major effect on the way Americans built and maintained their homes. As noted by the Centers for Disease Control and Prevention and U.S. Department of Housing and Urban Development (2006), the high cost of heating and cooling homes required action, but some of the actions taken were ill advised or failed to consider healthy housing concerns. Sealing buildings for energy efficiency and using off-gassing building materials containing urea-formaldehyde, vinyl, or new glues created toxic environments. These newly sealed environments were not refreshed with air; the resultant accumulation of both chemical and biologic pollutants and moisture led to mold growth, representing new threats to both short- and long-term health. The results of these actions are still being dealt with today.

The first to take code action was the American Society of Heating, Refrigerating, and Air-Conditioning Engineers with the publication of 90-75: *Energy Conservation in New Building Design* (1975). Model energy codes were more thoroughly developed in the early 1980s as a direct result of the energy crises and the knowledge that a huge portion of energy demands are from buildings, both residential and commercial. These energy codes followed the previous energy efficiency guidelines and made an attempt to overlay the engineering model for energy use onto the Building Code. Initially, this was an imperfect fit for two reasons. There was no mandate at the national or state level to encourage or require adoption of these codes; they were model codes offered for a jurisdiction to adopt by choice. Those who did adopt these codes had a breaking-in period while inspectors, with limited engineering and energy backgrounds, learned the code and enforcement methods. Regulating energy conservation was outside the traditional role of structural, fire, and life safety inspections.

These early versions of a model energy code led to a more consolidated energy conservation enforcement tool, the International Energy Conservation Code (IECC), in 1998. The IECC represented a joining of the disparate code organizations to agree on a set of energy efficiency minimums. The IECC regulates the overall energy efficiency of the structure and seeks to reduce the energy needed to maintain a healthy, comfortable, and fully functioning indoor environment (Department of Energy 2010). The code applies to much of the structure, such as walls, floors, ceilings, doors, windows, heating, ventilating, cooling, lighting, and water heating.

GREEN BUILDING IS BORN

Green building did not descend from the Building Code but rather evolved around it. During the last several decades, there has been increased awareness of the human effect on the environment. As the population increases in a nation, there is a corresponding increase in demand for raw materials and in accumulation of waste. In areas with low population density, this effect is not as clear as it is in higher-density areas. This is probably why Europe has been the vanguard of clean energy, environmental protection, and energy-efficient houses. As the United States has grown in population, it has become more evident that clean air, water, and soil matter. Building green in most places is voluntary (but that may be changing— Boulder, Colorado; Washington, DC; Austin, Texas, and many other jurisdictions mandate many green building practices).

Environmental awareness is not new (Henry David Thoreau wrote *Walden Pond* in 1854, John Muir formed the Sierra Club in 1892, and Aldo Leopold's *A Sand County Almanac* was published in 1949), but it has gained more prominence. Earth Day became an unofficial holiday on April 22, 1970. The Clean Air Act, Clean Water Act, and Endangered Species Act all were passed in the 1970s. Green building grew despite the downplay of conservation urgency as many smaller problems became apparent: deforestation in the Pacific Northwest and tropics; moldy houses that made people sick and rotted before they were paid off; and houses that were downright uncomfortable to be in (too hot, cold, damp, or dry).

Those who created green homes focused on health aspects and energy conservation from the start. As mentioned earlier, when houses were built tighter for energy conservation, concerns grew about volatile organic compounds off-gassing from various building materials and products. Formaldehyde adhesive in plywood is one example. Green builders and designers introduced concepts that included maintaining an adequate supply of fresh air and eliminating noxious fumes and odors with exhaust ventilation.

There are many definitions of green building, and probably the most oft-asked question is "What does green building really mean?" The most practical approach for builders, architects, and consumers may be to look at the various green rating systems and choose one that aligns with their particular interests or concerns. The U.S. Green Building Council's Leadership in Energy and Environmental Design and the National Green Building Standard are the two major green building programs in the United States (http://www.greenbuildingadvisor.com/ratings). Both are point-based systems that rate houses in a number of categories, including water and energy efficiency, resource conservation, and indoor air quality. Because they have wider publicity, national programs tend to have better name recognition than smaller local programs. Local and regional programs, however, are usually better tailored to local conditions and may be more appealing to home buyers (http://www.greenbuildingadvisor.com/green-basics/local-green-building-programs).

The two major green building programs have stark differences in how they were developed: The National Green Building Standard, because it is a standard approved by the American National Standards Institute, was developed through a consensus process that includes broad stakeholder representation (http://www.greenbuildingadvisor.com/ngbs). The Leadership in Energy and Environmental Design, developed by the U.S. Green Building Council, considered input from many parties, yet did not pass through a formal consensus process (http://www.greenbuildingadvisor.com/green-basics/leed-homes). Because many green programs are developed outside the standard consensus model, they can promote more aggressive practices than what a minimum standard or building code could specify. In fact, people may ask, if green building is watered down into a consensus standard, is it still green? As green building works its way into the code books, "light green" will become standard practice, "deep green" will become slightly better practice, and extreme green (e.g., the Living Building Challenge; http://www.ilbi.org/the-standard) will become less extreme and gain wider acceptance.

Whatever the program or definition, at its core, green building means doing less harm to the environment in the process of home building and not making people sick after they move into a house. This can be done by efficiently designing and building houses that will last, that will use less water and energy, and that are healthy to live in.

Green homes are not only comfortable and affordable to live in but also pleasing to move through because of the natural light, fresh air, and open spaces. Well-designed rooms make people feel good; they are more productive and happy in green buildings. Making good use of day lighting, ventilation, and pleasing aesthetics encourages workers to be more productive in the workplace, students to be more productive in school, and homeowners to be happier at home (Wilson

1999). Despite the evidence, some have questioned whether green homes are indeed healthy. The National Center for Healthy Housing compared major national green building guidelines with its own set of recommended healthy housing criteria to determine whether these programs adequately protect residents from housing conditions known to affect health status (Morley and Tohn 2008). The results showed that although all the programs have components aimed at improving resident health, many are missing critical elements. For example, protection from contaminants such as lead, radon, and pesticides are not uniformly covered. The report suggests ways to strengthen the occupant health criteria for green building programs so they can deliver even greater benefits to the families who reside in them.

There is another aspect central to green building that is not typically mentioned: The house should look good and be comfortable. Why? Because people take care of things they like, and when you take care of things, they tend to last. Many believe that green houses are better houses—you can build a high-quality house that is not green, but you cannot build a green house that is not high quality. Many houses are beautiful but not comfortable or energy efficient, and many comfortable and efficient houses are not especially beautiful. Houses that look good and are comfortable have a high level of design involved, and through meticulous planning and design, most of the other goals of green building are achieved: minimizing waste, maximizing efficiency, making sure the indoor air is clean, and choosing materials that tread lightly on local and global ecosystems. Green building takes a systems approach to building and remodeling houses. As noted earlier, partial improvements can do more harm than good. Tight houses can cause indoor air-quality problems, such as "sick building syndrome." Controlled mechanical ventilation is necessary with tighter houses, making them more energy efficient with indoor air quality superior to that of a leaky old house. Beyond indoor air quality, green building delivers better houses, inspected to verify adherence to standards throughout construction. The design process often incorporates better engineering to optimize systems that lower cost and increase performance. Green building also encourages sub-trades to work together to achieve high-performance homes.

GREEN AND EFFICIENT HOMES TAKE LESS

By its very nature, home building is disruptive to the site: You scrape away the topsoil, dig a very big hole, cut down many of the existing trees and shrubs, and sometimes replace them with non-native plants. Birds, bees, foxes, and trees are displaced in the process, and often they do not return, but it does not have to be this way. Some houses give as much as they take; many houses could give more and take less. Storm water runoff is a good example. Houses on small lots (less than one eighth of an acre), such as those in a city, can have two thirds of their land surface covered with impervious surfaces—roof, driveway, walkway, and patio. Houses in suburban neighborhoods with quarter-acre lots can steal approximately 40% of the absorptive surface area. This translates into a great deal of land shedding water rather than absorbing it. When rainwater absorbs into the ground, it recharges ground water supplies. Also, the ground cleans the water on the way down so that clean drinking water can be pumped out. When rainwater sheds from lots, it takes pet waste, pesticides, and fertilizers from lawns, as well as oil, gas, and grease from driveways. All of this water is washed into storm drains and dumped into rivers and lakes, overloading city sewer systems, polluting rivers and lakes, and poisoning aquatic plant and animal life. Because the water was not cleaned naturally by the soil, money must be spent on energy for water-treatment plants to clean it for drinking water. All in all, this is a bad buy. Vegetative roofs are one example of how a home can reduce the amount of rainwater that is directed into the sewer system, and they can provide a home or food for birds and bees. Smaller houses are another example of how houses can take less and give back more. Small houses have a smaller footprint (which disturbs the site less, meaning less storm water runoff and fewer trees removed from the site), use less materials (which means fewer trees to cut down to make the lumber), and are typically more energy efficient (which gives back to the occupants and the earth, and makes them cleaner and less expensive).

Storm water runoff and native plants are examples of local environmental issues, but houses can affect the global environment too. The framing lumber we use often comes from the other side of the country. Siding materials and steel pipes are often shipped across the ocean. Hardwoods for cabinetry and floors frequently come from tropical rain forests that are increasingly becoming deserts. Using less material to build houses and making smarter choices about which material to use can alleviate environmental problems. Begin by using less. For example, one way to use less wood when building a house is to switch from placing studs, joists, and rafters 16 inches apart to placing them 24 inches apart. This is variously known as optimum value engineering or advanced framing (for more information see http://www.greenbuildingadvisor.com/efficient-framing). This practice can reduce lumber by at least one third with no negative effect on structural integrity (and it is allowed in the IRC). You can also save wood by designing houses a little smarter: because sheets of plywood come in 4-foot widths, it makes sense to design walls and roofs to take advantage of these increments. Similarly, placing window and door openings where studs fall on layout, rather than adding extra studs to accommodate them, saves a significant amount of lumber. Taken together, these improvements can decrease lumber use by 40%. Eliminating extraneous wood also improves the energy efficiency of a roof or wall, as more room is made for insulation.

We can do less harm to global environments by choosing local materials when possible. This helps discourage rainforest destruction and cuts greenhouse gasses by eliminating energy used in shipping steel pipe or cement siding. Globalization makes sense for some things, such as digital work, but it makes less and less sense for building materials. Is it greener to ship bamboo floors from China than it is to use locally grown oak? Probably not. One way to gauge the environmental effects of material choices is through life-cycle assessments, such as the "Building for Environmental and Economic Sustainability" tool (http://www.bfrl.nist.gov/oae/software/bees), published by the National Institute of Standards and Technology, and the "Athena Institute Environmental Impact Estimator" (http://www.athenasmi.org/tools/impactEstimator). For more on life-cycle assessment, refer to "Life Cycle Assessment Is a Tool, Not a Silver Bullet" (http://www.greenbuildingadvisor.com/life-cycle).

Energy-efficient homes result from systems-thinking and smart tradeoffs. Energy efficiency begins with making good use of the sun—keeping heat out in the summer and letting it in during the winter while letting in daylight year round. Investing in better insulation and windows means that you can reduce the size of mechanical systems. These tradeoffs make a house cheaper to operate, but often they save money in the construction stage too. In fact, superinsulated houses can actually cost little or nothing extra to build because large mechanical systems are significantly reduced or eliminated altogether (http://www.greenbuildingadvisor.com/homes/first-us-passive-house-shows-energy-efficiency-can-be-affordable).

Using less water is also important in green building. This can be accomplished through efficient plumbing and wastewater systems, as well as using water-saving fixtures and appliances. These water-saving features often save energy by reducing the amount of hot water needed. Also, municipalities pump less water to homes that use less water; a municipality's energy savings is not reflected on the water bill, but homeowners may save on property tax instead.

There are a few ways to benchmark energy use in homes. Energy Star is the most well known. The Energy Star Homes program (http://www.energystar.gov/index.cfm?c=bldrs_lenders_raters.pt_bldr) is run by the U.S. Environmental Protection Agency (EPA). The program is limited in scope compared with green-building certification systems, but it remains an important benchmark for energy efficiency and is cited in other rating guidelines. Energy Star homes are at least 15% more energy efficient than a home that barely meets the 2004 IRC. According to the EPA, an Energy Star house is typically 20% to 30% more energy efficient than a conventionally built house. To promote water conservation in new homes, the EPA has launched a companion program to Energy Star called WaterSense (http://www.epa. gov/watersense). Another companion program, Indoor airPLUS (http://www.epa. gov/indoorairplus), includes specifications designed to lower risks for indoor mold, radon, combustion gases, and toxic chemicals. The program mandates more than 30 design and construction features beyond Energy Star requirements.

At the other end of the energy use spectrum is the Passive House Standard. This standard is the highest level of energy conservation. In central Europe, Passiv-Haus requires that a building follow these requirements:

- The building must not use more than 15 kWh/m² per year in heating and cooling energy;
- the total energy consumption (energy for heating, hot water, and electricity) must not be more than 42 kWh/m² per year; and
- the total primary energy (e.g., source energy for electricity) consumption must not be more than 120 kWh/m² per year.

It is true that getting a green rating will not guarantee energy efficiency (although some do, such as Environments for Living; see http://www.greenbuilding advisor.com/green-basics/environments-living) or healthful air quality, as various rating programs weigh components differently. That is why it is important to research the different systems and choose one that aligns with your particular needs. Also, at the end of the day, houses are designed and built by people. Mistakes made in the building or design process can sabotage a structure's performance; thus architects and builders must understand the building science involved with tightly built houses. Each part affects the others. For example, a builder may use a peel-and-stick waterproof membrane instead of number 30 felt paper as an underlayment for roofing materials. This substitution changes the direction that the roof assembly can dry if it gets wet—it can only dry inward. Other problems can occur after the house is completed: A homeowner may choose to put up vinyl wallpaper that is impermeable to moisture. If there is an impermeable layer anywhere else in the wall assembly, it can trap moisture and cause mold growth. Home design and modification must be weighed carefully to avoid harmful unintended consequences.

HOUSES SHOULD LAST A LONG TIME

The cost of durability is spread over the life of a house. The longer a house lasts, the longer the period of time over which the environmental consequences of its construction will be spread out. Some houses built in the 1980s and 1990s rotted away after 12 years. This is extremely bad amortization of environmental costs. Similarly, tearing down a perfectly good house to build a new one is a bad environmental buy.

The house's enclosure should hold up to the elements—houses should be able to withstand rainfall, humidity, heavy snowfall, hail, flooding, and intense sun. This requires a basic understanding of building science, particularly water management. It also means choosing materials that will hold up for a long time. Many of the things that make houses last, such as flashing details, vapor control, and groundwater management, are part of the building code. You can always do better than code minimum, and green building embraces that idea. One example is roof overhangs that can protect siding and windows from rainwater, thus extending their life and making them less susceptible to leaks. The IRC does not require roof overhangs, but many green rating programs award extra points for them. Durability also encompasses houses that will be around for a long time because the people like them or continue to find ways to use their features. Timeless design, accessibility, and adaptability are all important. If interior spaces can be reconfigured easily with little actual construction, future alterations will be less expensive, environmental burdens will be lower, and the house will be more livable.

CONCLUSION

This chapter has described what a green home is: durable, efficient, and healthful to live in. Green homes take less from the environment while giving more back. One of the biggest challenges that builders, remodelers, and architects cite is building code and code officials. Are green homes against the law? No. Many green and healthy construction techniques have been mandated by the IRC and are part of the newest version of the IRC. However, the perception of best practices being against the code lingers. For example, sealed crawlspaces are a building science best practice, and the IRC has just recently caught up with this practice. Nevertheless, ventilated crawlspaces are so ingrained into the way people build houses that many never noticed the recent upgrade. Before the new version of the code, builders had trouble convincing their local inspector that a sealed crawlspace was a good idea.

With green building working its way into the building code, does that mean the world is safe from global warming, pollution, and asthma? Not really. Although it is important that new houses are significantly healthier and more energy efficient than older houses, there are many more leaky old houses in disrepair than tight new ones in good condition. The real solution is in retrofitting existing houses to be tight, healthy, and safe houses. For all homes, the last part of the equation is to help residents understand the principles of healthy homes (see Chapters 2 and 3).

Green building and building codes both aim for the same general target: better houses. In this way, building codes and green building practices share the same spirit: safe, healthful spaces that do not waste energy and that are durable. As green building works its way into the code books, the definition of green will move further toward what is considered deep green or extreme green today. Green building is a better way to build and remodel houses, generating homes that are energy efficient, healthful to live in, and long lasting, making them a good amortization of natural resources. Green building represents the next step in quality.

REFERENCES

Centers for Disease Control and Prevention and U.S. Department of Housing and Urban Development. *Healthy Housing Reference Manual.* Atlanta, GA: Centers for Disease Control and Prevention and U.S. Department of Housing and Urban Development, 2006. Available at: http://www.cdc.gov/nceh/publications/books/housing/housing.htm.

Department of Energy. *Building Energy Codes 101—An Introduction* (2010). Available at: http://www.energycodes.gov/training/pdfs/codes_101.pdf. Accessed March 26, 2010.

Mood, E. *Housing and Health: APHA-CDC Recommended Minimum Housing Standards.* Washington, DC: American Public Health Association, 1986.

Morley, R., and E. Tohn. *How Healthy Are National Green Building Programs?* Columbia, MD: National Center for Health Housing, 2008. Available at: http://www.nchh.org/Policy/Policy-Projects/Green-Building-Analysis.aspx. Accessed March 11, 2010.

Wilson, A. Daylighting: Energy and productivity benefits. *Environmental Building News,* September 1999.

Fire Prevention Personnel

Shane Diekman, PhD, MPH, and
Mark Jackson, BS, REHS

Fire prevention personnel—firefighters and trained non-firefighters—often work to create healthier homes by participating in community education, training, and home visits. This chapter describes what fire prevention personnel should look for during home visit assessments. It also explains how they can use simple prevention strategies, such as smoke alarm installation and prevention education, to improve the safety of homes. Although this chapter focuses on fire prevention, it also touches on other home injury prevention topics, such as scald burns and carbon monoxide poisoning.

In addition, the chapter highlights the Smoke Alarm Installation and Fire Safety Education (SAIFE) program instituted by the Centers for Disease Control and Prevention (CDC). This program is an example of an established approach that incorporates both environmental change (smoke alarms) and prevention education. The chapter also presents materials from the CDC's *Fire Safe Seniors Toolkit* that illustrate the practical application of home fire safety assessments and corresponding education.

THE HOME FIRE PROBLEM

Fire Statistics

The United States has the eighth highest fire death rate of all industrialized countries (International Association for the Study of Insurance Economics 2009). Deaths from fires and burns are the sixth most common cause of unintentional injury deaths in the United States (CDC 2006). In 2008, approximately 515,000 fires occurred in structures, and 78% (n = 403,000) of these fires occurred in homes[1] (Karter 2009). These home fires resulted in an estimated 13,560 civilian injuries, 2,755 civilian deaths, and $8.6 billion in direct property damage (Karter 2009). The number of home fires and fire-related injuries and deaths has gradually declined over the past 30 years, with a relative plateau since 1999 (Ahrens 2009; Flynn 2008). Still, home fires remain a public health problem with substantial implications for individuals and society. Fortunately, many home fires and their associated consequences are preventable.

Leading Causes of Home Fires, Injuries, Deaths, and Property Damage

According to the National Fire Protection Association (NFPA), cooking is the leading cause of home fires and injuries, smoking materials are the leading cause of death, and heating equipment fires cause the largest percentage of direct property damage (Ahrens 2010). Following are the leading causes of home structure fires, injuries, deaths, and property damage using 2003–2007 data (adapted from Ahrens 2010). These statistics are based on fires that were reported to the fire department and exclude those handled without fire department assistance.

- The leading causes of home *fires* are
  - cooking equipment (40%),
  - heating equipment (18%),
  - intentionally setting a fire (8%),
  - electrical distribution and lighting equipment (6%),
  - smoking materials (5%),
  - clothes dryer or washer (4%),
  - candle (4%), and
  - playing with heat source (2%).
- The leading causes of home fire *injuries* are
  - cooking equipment (36%),
  - heating equipment (13%),
  - candle (10%),
  - smoking materials (10%),
  - intentionally setting a fire (7%),
  - electrical distribution and lighting equipment (7%),
  - playing with heat source (6%), and
  - clothes dryer or washer (3%).

---

[1] The term "homes" was a subset of the broader category of residential fires and included one- and two-family dwellings, duplexes, manufactured homes, apartments, townhouses, rowhouses, and condominiums. Residential properties excluded from this definition were hotels and motels, college dormitories, residential board and care or assisted living, unclassified residential properties, and boarding houses.

- The leading causes of home fire *deaths* are
  - smoking materials (25%),
  - heating equipment (22%),
  - cooking equipment (17%),
  - electrical distribution and lighting equipment (12%),
  - intentionally setting a fire (12%),
  - candle (6%), and
  - playing with heat source (4%).
- The leading causes of home fire *property damage* are
  - heating equipment (13%),
  - cooking equipment (11%),
  - electrical distribution and lighting equipment (11%),
  - intentionally setting a fire (9%),
  - candle (7%),
  - smoking materials (7%), and
  - playing with heat source (3%).

These data represent the leading causes of the fire problem at a national level. Local data will provide a better picture of the problem within a particular community and can often be obtained from fire departments. An even better way to determine household risk is to conduct home visit assessments, which are discussed later in this chapter. This approach allows prevention personnel to assess and address risk in real time.

Risk Factors

Many characteristics at the individual, home, and environmental levels increase the risk for home fires and associated injuries. Table 9.1 lists the main risk factors.

Fire safety knowledge and associated skills are also important factors in the overall safety of a home. However, there is a lack of studies relating these factors to outcomes such as fires and fire-related injuries. This research gap suggests the need for evidence-based approaches to education and behavior change.

Identifying risk factors for home fires and fire-related injuries and deaths helps guide efforts to improve these problems. Risk factors that cannot be modified, such as age and race, may identify the groups of individuals on whom to focus prevention efforts. Modifiable risk factors, such as smoking or home characteristics, are potential target areas for behavior or environmental changes.

Formative research and evaluations, such as community needs assessments, are important steps in designing prevention programs that meet community needs, address community strengths and weakness, and incorporate key issues.

TABLE 9.1—INDIVIDUAL, HOME, AND ENVIRONMENTAL RISK FACTORS FOR RESIDENTIAL FIRES AND ASSOCIATED INJURIES AND DEATHS

Environmental U.S. Census region • South • North Central Rural communities Poverty	
Individual Age • <5 years • ≥65 years Sex • Male Race and ethnicity • African American • Native American Physical or cognitive disabilities Behaviors • Tobacco smoking • Alcohol use • Other drug use, including medication Low annual income Low educational attainment	Home Absence of working smoke alarms Lack of residential sprinklers Poor housing stock (e.g., mobile or manufactured home) Age of home (>20 years) Lack of telephone Lack of home ownership Lack of ignition-resistant household materials (e.g., mattress, furniture)

Adapted from Flynn, J.D. Characteristics of Home Fire Victims. Quincy, MA: National Fire Protection Association, Fire Analysis and Research Division, 2008. Warda, L., M. Tenenbein, and M.E.K. Moffatt. House fire injury prevention update. Part I. A review of risk factors for fatal and non-fatal house fire injury. Inj Prev 1999:5:145–50.

These activities should be conducted before implementing any prevention program so they can be incorporated into or inform its design. Fire prevention programs should create a community risk profile by identifying the fire safety problems in the community and the demographic characteristics of those people at risk. This information will identify the leading causes of community risks, where these problems are occurring, and who is being affected by the risk. It can also help inform the design and delivery of appropriate prevention strategies for the community.

The following section describes the traditional approaches to fire prevention and levels of evidence for specific interventions.

FIRE PREVENTION APPROACHES

Members of the fire service traditionally have focused their fire prevention efforts on the "Three E's": engineering, enforcement, and education. Together, these approaches have advanced fire prevention by preventing, controlling, and mitigating the impact of fires.

Engineering Approaches

Fire protection engineering applies science and engineering principles to fire-related situations or settings to identify risks and design safeguards to reduce those risks. In particular, technology is used to create safer products or modify the environment where the risk is occurring. Fire protection strategies and solutions include risk analyses, fire suppression systems (e.g., residential sprinklers), smoke alarms, building design and layout planning, fire modeling, and human behavior during fire events.

Enforcement Approaches

The NFPA develops, publishes, and disseminates consensus codes and standards designed to prevent fires and minimize the consequences during and after fire situations. These codes and standards are adopted at the state and local levels. Code enforcement is necessary to make sure that adopted standards of fire safety are being met in various settings. Fire inspectors are involved in the planning and building phases of residential structures to ensure that code regulations are being met. After a structure is built, fire inspectors conduct inspections to assess code compliance and areas where danger to life or property is possible. Code inspection and enforcement are mandatory for most commercial settings. Similarly, fire inspectors regularly visit group residential settings, such as nursing homes, college dormitories, and apartment complexes.

For various reasons, including time constraints, individual households are not routinely inspected for code compliance, which presents a challenge for fire prevention. Even though new construction will be built to code, these codes change over time to reflect technologic advances. Therefore, homes built before these changes will no longer be up to code without occupants taking action. In addition, the behavior of occupants can compromise fire safety by violating codes. For example, research indicates that occupants sometimes remove or disable smoke alarms when "nuisance" alarms go off too frequently.

Education Approaches

Most large, career fire departments, in which all members are compensated for their services, provide planned fire safety education to their community members. Fire safety education efforts are often part of larger fire prevention programs, which may include the distribution and installation of smoke alarms or campaigns to educate seniors about key safety topics. All programs tend to mix messages of general injury prevention, safety, fire prevention, and escape in case of a fire.

A main focus of fire prevention education is on educating elementary students through presentations in school settings. Firefighters often develop their own presentations on the basis of shared information from other fire departments and widely available resource materials from national organizations (e.g., the U.S. Fire Administration, NFPA, and Home Safety Council). In most cases the firefighters, as experts, are expected to present information in a manner that is appropriate for each age group. Yet, many fire safety messages can be delivered effectively by well-trained, non-fire service educators, especially if these presenters are using nationally recognized programs, such as NFPA's *Risk Watch*, *Learn Not to Burn*, or *Remembering When*. For example, many teachers across the United States incorporate the *Learn Not to Burn* program into their school curriculum.

When fire safety education is delivered in home environments, it provides a unique opportunity to address various risk factors present in the home at that moment. Following is an example of how all three approaches—engineering, enforcement, and education—provide different solutions for the same problem in a home setting.

Problem: A home inspection revealed that several smoke alarms were not working because the batteries were depleted.

Engineering solution:
- Hard-wire smoke alarms and alarm systems into home electrical systems; upgrade alarms with tamperproof, long-lasting lithium batteries.

Enforcement solution:
- Require updated smoke alarms and alarm systems, and enforce penalties for nonworking smoke alarms.

Education solution:
- Reinforce the importance of working smoke alarms by talking about how they decrease the risk of death in a home fire.

For home visits, education and simple environmental changes are the most viable options to reduce fire risk. Enforcement is generally not an option because most prevention personnel are not certified in code enforcement and the potential of fines would deter access to the homes that prevention personnel are trying to enter. When possible, residents should be educated about potential engineering solutions. However, some of these solutions, such as residential sprinklers, may only be viable when there is broader political and policy support and change. Therefore, the installation of long-lasting smoke alarms, coupled with fire safety education, remains fire prevention personnel's best option for reducing fire risk in a home. Ultimately, fire prevention program coordinators should determine which options can be addressed by the program.

Evidence for Fire Prevention Interventions

In the 2007 *Handbook of Injury and Violence Prevention*'s chapter "Interventions to Prevent Residential Fire Injury," Warda and Ballesteros identified existing fire-prevention interventions, which were categorized into products, behavioral interventions, and multilevel approaches. Each intervention was assessed to determine its current level of evidence (i.e., effective, promising, insufficient evidence, no evidence, harmful). Following is a summary of the interventions that were identified as effective or promising.

Products:
- smoke alarms (effective)
- child-resistant lighters (effective)
- fire-safe cigarettes (promising)
- ignition-resistant household materials (promising)

Behavioral interventions:
- community-societal interventions, including legislation (promising)

Multilevel approaches:
- smoke alarm installation (effective) and distribution (promising)

There is insufficient evidence that education by itself reduces fire risk or fire-related injuries. However, education contributes to the effectiveness of multifactorial strategies, particularly those that involve behavior change, such as strategies to increase smoke alarm use and function. When educational approaches are used, they should be evidence-based and guided by the principles of teaching, learning, and behavior change to increase their likelihood of success. Legislative interventions, which are often designed to influence behaviors and actions of individuals, also rely on education to increase acceptance and adoptability (Shaw and Ogolla 2006).

As fire-prevention programs are developed and refined, the available evidence for certain fire-prevention strategies should be considered. The Warda and Ballesteros chapter suggests that several effective and promising strategies can be addressed during home visits, including smoke alarms, child-resistant lighters, and fire-safe cigarettes.

Smoke alarms—more specifically, smoke alarm installation programs—seem to be the most effective fire-prevention strategy.

Smoke alarms are effective, reliable, and inexpensive devices that provide early warning during residential fires. Smoke alarms decrease the risk of death in a home fire by up to 50% (Ahrens 2004). In 2003–2006, 63% of reported home fire deaths resulted from fires in homes with no smoke alarms or no working smoke alarms (Ahrens 2009). Estimates consistently indicate that more than 90% of U.S. households report having at least one smoke alarm (NFPA 2008; U.S. Census Bureau 2007). However, approximately one quarter of U.S. households lack working smoke alarms, and those households least likely to have an alarm often include people at a higher risk of being injured in a fire (Harvey et al. 1998). In fact, most high-risk groups for residential fire fatality—the poor, seniors, heavy drinkers, households with less than high school education, and those in rural areas and the southern United States—are less likely to have smoke alarms (Warda and Ballesteros 2007).

An established strategy to increase smoke alarm use among high-risk households is the direct installation of smoke alarms by trained individuals, such as firefighters (Ballesteros et al. 2005; Harvey et al. 2004). Most recommendations call for working smoke alarms on every level of the home and inside and outside of each sleeping area.[2]

Although the proper installation of smoke alarms helps to protect households in the event of a fire, education must focus on testing and maintenance. In addition, occupants should plan and practice their escape to further ensure a safe exit should a fire occur. Education is also an important component of home visits because many risk factors can be modified with appropriate knowledge and behavior change. For example, occupants may need to be educated on how to acquire, install, test, and maintain a smoke alarm or how to develop, practice, and implement a fire escape plan (Thompson, Waterman, and Sleet 2004).

Fire prevention programs that include home visits offer considerable promise because they can assess and address the specific risks in each home. Although these efforts can be time consuming, they offer tremendous prevention potential. Following is a description of a well-established smoke alarm installation and fire safety education program.

---

[2] For even better protection, smoke alarms can be interconnected. The value of interconnected smoke alarms is that when one alarm sounds, they all do. There are two types of interconnected smoke alarms: hard-wired (into the electrical system) and wireless. Whether smoke alarms are hard-wired or wireless, all interconnected smoke alarms must be compatible with one another, as specified by the manufacturer. A licensed electrician may be needed to replace existing hard-wired smoke alarms with those capable of wireless interconnection.

The Centers for Disease Control and Prevention's *Smoke Alarm Installation and Fire Safety Education* Program

Since 1998, the CDC has funded smoke alarm installation programs and fire safety education programs in high-risk communities with fire death rates higher than state and national averages and median household incomes below the poverty level. In addition, SAIFE programs target households with children (age ≤ 5 years) and older adults (age ≥ 65 years). As of March 2010, program staff had enrolled 249,724 high-risk homes, installed 487,827 long-lasting smoke alarms, and estimated that 3,143 lives potentially had been saved. A potential life saved was defined as a situation in which a program-installed smoke alarm was the initial warning to the resident(s) that there was smoke or fire in the home. The SAIFE Program currently is delivered through 13 state health departments, 3 large city fire departments, and 1 children's hospital. For more information about the SAIFE program, visit the CDC's website at http://www.cdc.gov/ncipc/factsheets/fireactivities.htm.

The Centers for Disease Control and Prevention *Fire Safe Seniors* Toolkit

In 2006, the CDC partnered with the Meals on Wheels Association of America (MOWAA) to develop and implement the Residential Fire Homebound Elderly Lifeline Project (Fire H.E.L.P.). Fire H.E.L.P. was designed to promote residential fire safety among homebound older adults, with the goal of reducing injuries and loss of property and life caused by fire and fire-related hazards. Fire H.E.L.P. consists of three major components: conducting home assessments; providing education on fire risk factors and the importance of smoke alarms and escape planning; and partnering with local fire departments to install free smoke alarms with long-life lithium batteries. The CDC provided technical assistance to MOWAA by developing a Fire H.E.L.P. train-the-trainer toolkit and training MOWAA staff to use it. In 2009, the CDC adapted the Fire H.E.L.P. toolkit and created the *Fire Safe Seniors Toolkit*. The new toolkit was designed to provide community-based organizations with instructional curricula about how to implement the program, a home assessment tool to determine smoke alarm needs, and education materials to increase client knowledge about fire safety. For more information about CDC's *Fire Safe Seniors Toolkit*, visit http://www.cdc.gov/HomeandRecreationalSafety/Fire-Prevention/index.html.

Two main features of the CDC SAIFE program and the *Fire Safe Seniors Toolkit* are home safety assessment and the delivery of fire safety education. Prevention programs can use checklists to assess the safety of home environments. These checklists should be designed so that the person filling them out can take action (e.g., education, environmental modification) to address identified risk factors.

HOME SAFETY CHECKLISTS

Table 9.2 contains a home safety checklist that covers the main fire (and related) risk factors in most homes, factors that can be easily identified through observation or by asking the occupant (Table 9.2).

In most cases, fire prevention personnel will be able to identify and address only a few risk factors during a home visit. These areas should be determined on the basis of research about the target audience and the program goals. The primary purpose of the *Fire Safe Seniors Toolkit* checklist is to assess the presence of working smoke alarms in the house and selected injury-related risk factors (e.g., clutter that increases both fire and fall risks). The goal of the program is to determine whether a household has working smoke alarms on every level of the home and outside of every sleeping area. Table 9.3 contains a home fire safety checklist from the *Fire Safe Seniors Toolkit* illustrating how a few topics are selected and assessed. It should be noted that the *Fire Safe Seniors Toolkit* recommends smoke alarms (1) on every level of the home, including the basement, and (2) outside every sleeping area. These locations correspond to the minimum requirements found in NFPA 72, National Fire Alarm Code, at the time of the *Toolkit*'s original development. The most current edition of NFPA 72, National Fire Alarm and Signaling Code, recommends smoke alarms in every bedroom; larger homes may need additional smoke alarms installed throughout. Fire prevention program coordinators should research state laws and local ordinances about smoke alarm standards and recommended procedures to make sure they are compliant.

PREVENTION EDUCATION MESSAGES

If possible, the identified risk factors should be addressed during the home visit. Follow-up visits may be required for some home modifications or if identified risk factors are documented for referral purposes (e.g., installation of carbon monoxide detector devices or removal of clutter). At a minimum, occupants should be educated about the risk factors identified from the home safety checklist. Table 9.4 lists home safety education messages for each of the risk factors listed in the home safety checklist. These messages were compiled from the NFPA, U.S. Fire Administration, Home Safety Council, and CDC's National Center for Environmental Health fact sheets and websites.

The *Fire Safe Seniors Toolkit* fire safety education form was designed to make sure at least two risk factors are addressed during each home visit (Table 9.5). At a minimum, each client is educated about smoke alarms and escape plans. The form

TABLE 9.2—HOME FIRE SAFETY CHECKLIST

Smoke Alarms:
- ☐ Have you installed a smoke alarm outside every sleeping area and in every bedroom on each floor?
- ☐ Do you test your smoke alarm(s) every month?
- ☐ Do you replace the battery in your smoke alarm every year?
- ☐ Do you maintain your smoke alarms according to the manufacturer's recommendations?

Fire Escape Plan:
- ☐ Does your family have a fire escape plan prepared?
- ☐ Is your escape plan posted and regularly practiced?
- ☐ Do you know two ways out of each room in your home?
- ☐ Do you have a designated meeting place for everyone to go outside?
- ☐ Are emergency response numbers posted on all telephones?
- ☐ Do all family members know how to dial 911 for fire, police, or medical emergencies?
- ☐ Do you show your babysitter/guests your home escape routes and review 911 with her or him?
- ☐ Does your family (and babysitter) know the first rule in fire emergencies: GET OUT AND STAY OUT!!

Smoking Habits:
- ☐ Are all matches and lighters kept out of children's reach?
- ☐ Is "NO SMOKING IN BED" a rule of the house?
- ☐ Is your family aware that ash trays should NEVER be emptied into wastebaskets?
- ☐ Are there plenty of large, deep, sturdy ash trays throughout the house?

Cooking Safety:
- ☐ Do you stay in the kitchen when frying, grilling, or broiling food?
- ☐ Do you keep things that can easily catch fire (wooden spoons, oven mitts, towels) away from your stove top?
- ☐ Do you wear short, close-fitting, or tightly rolled sleeves when cooking?
- ☐ Do you have a 3-foot "kid-free zone" around the stove where hot food is being prepared?

Heating Safety:
- ☐ Do you keep anything that can burn 3 feet away from heating equipment, such as a fireplace, furnace, wood stove, and portable heaters?
- ☐ Do you use your oven for heating?
- ☐ Do you maintain your heating equipment and chimneys by having a qualified professional inspect them annually?
- ☐ Do you turn portable heaters off when you leave the room or go to bed?

Electrical Safety:
- ☐ Are appliances checked periodically for good operating conditions?
- ☐ Are you careful not to run extension cords under rugs or over hooks and nails?
- ☐ Do the electrical outlets in your bathroom have ground fault circuit interrupters installed?
- ☐ Are electrical outlets overloaded?
- ☐ Do all electrical outlets and switch covers have faceplates?

TABLE 9.2—(CONTINUED)

Children and Fire:
☐ Do you keep all lighters and matches stored away from children?
☐ Do you use only child-resistant lighters?
☐ Do your children know to tell an adult if they see matches or lighters?

Candle Safety:
☐ Do you blow out all candles when leaving the room or go to bed?
☐ Do you keep candles at least 12 inches away from anything that can burn?
☐ Are your candle holders sturdy and not easily tipped over?
☐ Do you use flashlights instead of candles during power outages?

Fire Extinguishers:
☐ Do you have approved fire extinguishers from an independent testing laboratory?
☐ Have you been trained by qualified personnel in how to operate and properly use your fire extinguisher?
☐ Do you have your fire extinguishers stored close to an exit?

Carbon Monoxide (CO) Safety:
☐ Do you have CO alarms installed on every level of your home and a central location outside each sleeping area?
☐ Do you test your CO alarm once per month?
☐ Does your CO alarm have a label of a recognized testing laboratory?
☐ Do you know what to do if your CO alarm sounds?

Scald/Burn Safety:
☐ Is your hot water heater set to a temperature of $\leq 120°F$?
☐ Do you use back burners and turn pot handles to the back of the stove when cooking?
☐ Do you keep hot foods and liquids away from table and counter edges?
☐ Do you cover all unused electrical outlets with safety devices?

Source: Checklist based on information from the National Fire Prevention Association, the U.S. Fire Administration, the Home Safety Council, and the Centers for Disease Control and Prevention's National Center for Environmental Health.

was designed to give the fire safety educator flexibility to deliver a range of messages on the basis of the needs and abilities of the resident; if appropriate, messages are also delivered about smoking, cooking, and alternative heating sources. Print materials are left behind to provide information about topics and messages not covered during the client education session and to reinforce delivered messages.

Another resource, the Home Safety Council website, includes a tool that generates a home safety checklist and corresponding prevention messages. You can access the generator online at http://www.homesafetycouncil.org/SafetyGuide/sg_checklistgenerator_w001.asp. The Home Safety Council, a national nonprofit

TABLE 9.3—FIRE SAFE SENIORS HOME ASSESSMENT TOOL

Date: _____ / _____ / _____
Assessor:_____
Client Name: _____
Client Address: _____
Zip: _____
Client Phone: (_____)_____   GENDER: ___M ___F
ETHNICITY (Circle one):   Caucasian   African American   Hispanic   Asian/Pacific Islander
                            Native American   Other:_____
Client Date of Birth: _____ / _____ / _____

Look for Smoke Alarms: • On every level of the home • Outside of every sleeping area	Alarm Status AM (alarm missing) NLB (non-lithium or unknown battery) NWL (non-working lithium alarm) >10 (working lithium alarm > 10 years old) OK (working lithium alarm < 10 years old)
Outside of sleeping area #1 Indicate level of home:_____	
Outside of sleeping area #2 Indicate level of home:_____	
Outside of sleeping area #3 Indicate level of home:_____	
Additional level of home without a sleeping area Indicate level of home:_____	
Additional level of home without a sleeping area Indicate level of home:_____	
Other area:	
Total number of new alarms needed: (AM + NLB + NWL + > 10):	

Escape barriers observed:
___Clutter hindering escape route
___Furniture blocking exit doors
___Security bars on doors or windows
___Windows nailed or painted shut
___Other:_____

Home ownership status:
___Client owns residence
___Client lives in residence occupied by owner or owned by family member
___Client rents residence

Number of people living in home: _____

TABLE 9.3—(CONTINUED)

LOOK FOR SMOKE ALARMS IN THE FOLLOWING LOCATIONS:
- ❏ On every level of the home, including the basement
- ❏ Outside of every sleeping area

THE FOLLOWING ALARMS SHOULD BE REPLACED
- ❏ Non-lithium battery alarms
- ❏ Alarms with unknown battery types
- ❏ Non-working lithium alarms
- ❏ Lithium alarms > 10 years old

Action Needed: **Smoke alarm installation**

Consent/waiver form signed by client: ____/____/____

Date alarm(s) installed: ____/____/____
Fire department (if applicable):_____

Date alarm(s) tested: ____/____/____
Alarm(s) tested by:_____

Source: This tool is based on the original version developed by the Centers for Disease Control and Prevention.

organization dedicated to preventing home-related injuries, is nationally recognized for its high-quality fire-prevention resources. Fire-prevention personnel can gain access to the Home Safety Council's content and tools by registering to become a member (at no charge) through the organization's main website.

The successful delivery of prevention messages requires training and practice. Following are a few tips (without training) for providing educational messages during home visits. These tips are based on the CDC's experience in working with these types of programs:

- Always combine an intervention (e.g., smoke alarm installation) with education. You cannot assume that people know how to maintain a smoke alarm or how to properly design a fire escape plan for their family and home.

- At a minimum, cover the most important topics and hit 2–3 primary messages you want the audience to remember. In home visits, there is often limited time and people may have limited retention. You want to make sure you identify your population's highest risk factors and drive home 2–3 simple messages that can reduce those risk factors.

TABLE 9.4 — FIRE SAFETY EDUCATION MESSAGES

Smoke Alarms:
- Install smoke alarms in every bedroom, outside each separate sleeping area, and on every level of the home, including the basement.
- Test your smoke alarms monthly by pushing the test button.
- Replace alkaline batteries in all smoke alarms at least once per year. If an alarm "chirps," warning the battery is low, replace the battery right away.
- Save the manufacturers' instructions for testing and maintenance purposes.
- Replace all smoke alarms, including alarms that use 10-year batteries and hard-wired alarms, when they are 10 years old, or sooner if they do not respond properly.

(Source: National Fire Protection Association)

Fire Escape Planning:
- Pull together everyone in your household and make a plan. Walk through your home and inspect all possible ways out of the home. Households with children should consider drawing a map of the home, marking two ways out of each room, including windows and doors. Practice your escape plan at least twice a year. Practice your plan at night too.
- Choose an outside meeting place (e.g., neighbor's house, a light post, mailbox, or stop sign) a safe distance in front of your home where everyone can meet after escaping. Make sure to mark the location of the meeting place on your escape plan.
- Have everyone memorize the emergency phone number of the fire department. That way, any member of the household can call from a neighbor's home or a cellular phone once safely outside.
- Tell guests or visitors to your home about your family's fire escape plan.
- Once you're out of the home, remember "Get out and stay out!" Never go back into a burning home.

(Source: National Fire Protection Association)

Smoking Safety:
- If you smoke, smoke outside.
- Never smoke in bed or if you have been drinking or taking medication.
- Before you throw out butts and ashes, make sure they are out by dousing in water or sand.
- Use large, deep, sturdy ashtrays, and place them on a flat surface.
- Keep matches and lighters away from children.
- Never smoke in a home where medical oxygen is being used.

(Source: National Fire Protection Association)

Cooking Safety:
- Stay in the kitchen when you are frying, grilling, or broiling food. If you leave the kitchen for even a short period of time, turn off the stove.

TABLE 9.4 — (CONTINUED)

• Keep anything that can catch fire — oven mitts, wooden utensils, food packaging, towels, or curtains — away from your stovetop.

• Wear short, close-fitting, or tightly rolled sleeves when cooking. Loose clothing can dangle onto stove burners and catch fire if it comes in contact with a gas flame or an electric burner.

• Have a "kid-free zone" of at least 3 feet around the stove and areas where hot food or drink is prepared or carried.

Heating Safety:

• Keep anything that can burn at least 3 feet away from heating equipment, such as the furnace, fireplace, wood stove, or portable heater.

• Never use your oven for heating.

• Maintain heating equipment and chimneys by having them cleaned and inspected annually by a qualified professional.

• Turn portable heaters off when leaving the room or going to bed. Consider buying portable heaters that turn off if they tip over.

Electrical Safety:

• Avoid running extension cords across doorways or under carpets.

• Replace or repair loose or damaged cords on all electrical devices.

• Make sure the electrical outlets in your bathroom have ground fault circuit interrupters installed.

• Do not overload your electrical outlets.

• Make sure all electrical outlets and switch covers have face plates.

Children and Fire Safety:

• Store all matches and lighters away from children, up high in a locked cabinet.

• Use only child-resistant lighters. Remember, child-resistant does not mean childproof.

• Make sure children know to tell an adult if they see matches or lighters.

• Make sure your children know what your smoke alarms sound like and know and practice your fire escape plan.

Candle Safety:

• Blow out all candles when leaving the room or going to bed.

• Keep candles a minimum of 12 inches away from anything that can burn.

• Use sturdy candle holders that are not easily tipped over.

• Do not use candles during power outages. Make sure you have a sufficient supply of flashlights and batteries.

TABLE 9.4—(CONTINUED)

Fire Extinguishers:

• Portable fire extinguishers have limited capacity to put out fires. Call the fire department if there is a fire. As a general rule, fire fighting should be left to the experts. Only use an extinguisher if you have been trained to do so.

• Choose a fire extinguisher that carries the label of an independent testing laboratory.

• Read the instructions that come with the fire extinguisher and become familiar with its parts and operation before a fire breaks out. Local fire departments or fire equipment distributors often offer hands-on fire extinguisher trainings.

• Install fire extinguishers close to an exit and keep your back to a clear exit when you use the device so that you can make an easy escape if the fire cannot be controlled. If the room fills with smoke, leave immediately.

• Before fighting a fire, be sure that everyone is leaving the building and someone has sounded the alarm or called the fire department.

• To operate a fire extinguisher, remember the word **PASS**:
  ○ **P**ull the pin. Hold the extinguisher with the nozzle pointing away from you, and release the locking mechanism.
  ○ **A**im low. Point the extinguisher at the base of the fire.
  ○ **S**queeze the lever slowly and evenly.
  ○ **S**weep the nozzle from side to side.

Carbon Monoxide (CO) Safety:

• Have CO alarms installed on every level of your home and in a central location outside each sleeping area.

• Test your CO alarm monthly.

• Purchase only CO alarms that have a label of a recognized testing laboratory.

• If the CO alarm sounds, immediately move to a fresh air location outdoors or by an open window or door. Make sure everyone inside the home is accounted for. Call for help from a fresh air location and stay there until emergency personnel arrive.

Scald/Burn Prevention:

• Never leave a child alone, especially in the bathroom or kitchen. If you must leave the room, take the child with you.

• Set your water heater thermostat to no higher than 120°F. Consider installing water faucets and shower heads containing anti-scald technology.

• Use back burners and turn pot handles to the back of the stove when cooking. Keep appliance cords out of children's reach, especially if the appliances contain hot foods or liquids. If you have young children, install tamper-resistant electrical receptacles. If replacement is not possible, cover unused electrical outlets with protective outlet covers.

• Keep hot foods and liquids away from table and counter edges. Never carry or hold children and hot foods or liquids at the same time. (Source: Safe Kids USA)

• If you burn yourself, cool the burn with cool water for 3–5 minutes. Seek medical help if needed.

TABLE 9.5—FIRE SAFE SENIORS CLIENT EDUCATION TOOL

Date: _____ / _____ / _____
Date of Birth: _____ / _____ / _____
Client Name:_____
Client Address:_____
Zip:_____
Client Phone: (_____)_____
Educator:_____
Client will be getting free smoke alarms (check one)   ☐ Yes   ☐ No

(NOTE: Obtain this information from client's file if you did not determine the eligibility yourself—do not ask client directly)

DISCUSSION OPENER: **"I would like to talk to you today about fire safety. Many older adults are injured or die each year because of home fires. If it's okay with you, I'd like to spend a few minutes discussing how you can prevent fires and what you can do in case of a fire. How does that sound?"**

If client agrees, continue with questions.
If client is not able or willing to have the discussion, check here:_____ and provide reason below:
Reason:_____

Discussion Questions and Messages *If client has limited attention span, discuss only main messages.* *Check understanding after each question.*	Topic Covered (✓)
1. IF CLIENT WILL GET SMOKE ALARMS (BUT DOES NOT YET HAVE THEM): • *Say:* **Smoke alarms will be installed for you soon.** • *Main message:* **Check your smoke alarms every month or ask someone to do it for you.** • *Message #2:* **Never disable your smoke alarm.** **IF CLIENT HAS ALREADY RECEIVED PROGRAM SMOKE ALARMS:** • *Say:* **I understand that some smoke alarms were recently installed for you.** • *Main message:* **Check your smoke alarms every month or ask someone to do it for you.** • *Message #2:* **Never disable your smoke alarm.** **IF CLIENT IS <u>NOT</u> ELIGIBLE FOR PROGRAM SMOKE ALARMS:** • *Ask:* **Do you have any smoke alarms?** • *IF YES:* **Check your smoke alarms every month or ask someone to do it for you. Never disable your smoke alarm.** • *IF NO:* **Smoke alarms can keep you safe in case of fire. Consider getting some installed in your home.**	

TABLE 9.5—(CONTINUED)

Discussion Questions and Messages *If client has limited attention span, discuss only main messages.* *Check understanding after each question.*	Topic Covered (✓)
2. Have you thought about how you might escape in case of fire? • *Main message:* **Plan your escape around your abilities.** • *Message #2:* If possible, identify two ways out of every room. • *Message #3:* Keep a phone and emergency numbers near your bed or sleeping area to call for help. • *Message #4:* If there is a fire, get out and stay out. • *Message #5:* If you can't get out, get as low to the ground as you can.	
3. Do you or anyone else who lives here smoke? • *Main message:* **Never smoke when you are lying down, drowsy, or in bed.** • *Message #2:* Use large, deep, sturdy ashtrays, and place them on a flat surface. • *Message #3:* Wet cigarette butts and ashes before emptying them into the trash.	
4. Do you ever use the stove to cook? • *Main message:* **Never leave food unattended on the stove.** • *Message #2:* Wear tight-fitting or rolled-up sleeves while cooking. • *Message #3:* Keep towels, curtains, and paper away from the stove.	
5. How do you stay warm when it gets cold outside? IF CLIENT USES A SPACE HEATER: • *Main message:* **Keep the space heater 3 feet away from anything that can burn, including you.** • *Message #2:* Unplug heaters when not in use, including when you leave your home or go to bed. • *Message #3:* Consider getting space heaters that automatically turn off if they tip over. IF CLIENT USES A FIREPLACE, WOOD STOVE, OR COAL STOVE: • *Main message:* **Have a professional clean and inspect your fireplace or stove once a year.** • *Message #2:* Do not burn green wood, artificial logs, boxes, or trash. • *Message #3:* Use a metal mesh fireplace screen to keep sparks inside. If your fireplace has glass doors, leave them open while burning a fire.	
HOW TO END THE DISCUSSION: • **Explain leave-behind materials.** • **Ask if client has any questions.** • **Thank client for his or her time.**	

TABLE 9.5—(CONTINUED)

Materials left with client	Quantity
Flyer about smoking, cooking, and heating safety	
Flyer about smoke alarms and escape planning	
Other:	
Other:	

Source: From the Fire Safe Seniors Toolkit developed by the Centers for Disease Control and Prevention.

- Tailor messages for each at-risk population (e.g., rural residents, older adults, children). Each group requires different messages depending on its needs and situation. For example, rural populations are primarily served by volunteer fire departments. Such populations need to know the location of and how to contact their local department. Some rural residents may not be on the 911 system and will need to know that it may take a department longer to respond to an emergency. Older adults need information tailored to their capabilities and needs. In addition, children and their parents may need specific education on safety regarding matches or lighters that other populations do not need.

- Capitalize on family interactions to promote safety messages. Parents can be an excellent source of safety messages for preschool-aged children if properly informed. Teach parents how to talk to their preschool-aged children about identifying potential dangers, such as hot items, or when to tell a grown-up about a danger or to ask for help. Conversely, children should be encouraged to discuss safety topics with their parents. For example, elementary school–aged children can remind parents to test smoke alarms or to practice a fire escape plan.

- Provide primary and secondary prevention messages. Both types of education are important so that people know what they can do to prevent fires or burns (primary prevention) and what to do in case a fire or burn occurs (secondary prevention). For example, a primary prevention message could tell an occupant never to leave food on a stove unattended while cooking, whereas a secondary prevention message would educate the occupant to slide a lid over a cooking pan to extinguish a fire if it occurs.

- When possible, enhance fire safety education messages by demonstrating the appropriate behaviors to the occupant. Even better, demonstrate the desired action and then have the occupant practice that behavior in front of you.

- Create easy-to-read print materials and translate them into the languages of your audience. A great resource for low-literacy education materials is found at the Home Safety Council website (http://www.homesafetycouncil.org/AboutUs/HSLP/hslp_literacy_w001.asp).

IMPORTANT CONSIDERATIONS

Many factors increase the success of home visit programs. The following section discusses some important issues to consider in developing, implementing, and evaluating programs to increase the safety of homes.

Training

Training is essential to the success of prevention activities because it develops skills and increases competence related to program goals, content, and strategies. In addition, the more individuals trained, the greater the potential program reach. Commonly mentioned barriers to training include time and cost, so it is important to address potential barriers as early as possible to increase the availability and success of training.

Fire prevention personnel need two separate sets of skills and knowledge to deliver education effectively. First, they need to be deeply familiar with the topic they are teaching (subject matter expertise). Second, they need to understand how best to transfer that information to the client (instructional expertise). Firefighters receive significant technical training about putting out fires, but transforming these skilled firefighters into fire prevention and safety educators requires training to hone communication skills and ensure consistency in message. For non-firefighters, training is even more important. It takes practice to become comfortable delivering key messages and recording important information onto standardized forms while establishing and maintaining rapport with clients.

As an example, the CDC created two versions of the train-the-trainer manuals for the *Fire Safe Seniors Toolkit*: a two-hour session for the client education piece and a four-hour session for both the home assessment and the client education pieces. Prevention program coordinators will need to determine their own training needs depending on the skills and experience of their trainers.

Partnerships

Partnerships are valuable resources to consider with any prevention program; partners can assist with program activities by committing time, money, skills, staffing, access to high-risk residents, and other resources. Factors that help partnerships achieve shared or complementary goals include trust, shared vision, investment, risk, responsibility, evaluation, management, and governance. Partnerships can be both beneficial and challenging, depending on the type of partnering organization. Prevention programs must weigh the potential benefits and challenges to determine whether a partnership is right in a specific situation. Before forming a partnership, programs should consider the different types of partnerships that may be appropriate for their situation. Following are the four main types of partnerships, which go from the least to the most intensive regarding the amount of time, level of trust, and sharing of turf:

Networking:
- This type of partnership provides a forum for the exchange of ideas and information for mutual benefit, often through newsletters, conferences, meetings, and electronic information sharing. It is one of the least formal forms of partnership.

Coordinating:
- This partnership involves exchanging information and altering activities for a common purpose.

Cooperating:
- This type of partnership involves exchanging information, altering activities, and sharing resources.

Collaborating:
- This kind of partnership includes enhancing the capacity of the other partner for mutual benefit and common purpose, in addition to the listed activities.

Table 9.6 shows examples of key fire prevention partners at the federal, national, state, and local levels. Although listed separately, many of these partners work closely together in fire prevention efforts.

TABLE 9.6—POTENTIAL PARTNERS

Federal/National	State	Local
Centers for Disease Control and Prevention	State Health Departments	Local Health Departments
U.S. Fire Administration	State Fire Marshall's Office	Local Fire Departments
National Fire Protection Association		Churches
Home Safety Council		Local Businesses
Safe Kids		Boy Scouts
Meals on Wheels Association of America		Local Meals on Wheels Programs

Follow-Up

It is extremely important to incorporate follow-up in any prevention activities. Follow-up activities can be a part of evaluation to assess program impacts or outcomes. Follow-up can also serve to take corrective action and reinforce messages that will make a home safer. For example, a follow-up assessment could indicate that a smoke alarm near the kitchen was disabled because the battery was removed. Prevention staff could document this (evaluation) and return the alarm to functioning status (corrective action). Prevention staff could also educate the occupant about the importance of keeping smoke alarms functional (reinforcement message). In addition, prevention staff could work with the occupant to determine the causes of the disabling. For example, perhaps the occupant did not know how to use the "hush" button during nuisance alarms, or perhaps the smoke alarm needs to be relocated to another area that reduces the likelihood of nuisance alarms.

CONCLUSION

Home visits provide an excellent opportunity for fire prevention personnel to improve home safety. Evidence suggests that smoke alarm installations are effective, reliable, and inexpensive means of decreasing the risk of death in a home fire by up to 50%. Home safety checklists can be devised to identify many of the fire and injury risk factors present in the home. In turn, trained fire prevention personnel can address these issues through education and simple environmental changes. Ultimately, it is up to fire prevention personnel to determine which options can be addressed by the program. However, smoke alarm installation programs seem to be the most effective intervention strategy, and can be augmented by education. The CDC's *Fire Safe Seniors Toolkit* offers a practical method of training fire prevention personnel to conduct home fire safety assessments and deliver targeted home safety education.

REFERENCES

Ahrens, M. *Home Structure Fires*. Quincy, MA: National Fire Protection Association, Fire Analysis and Research Division, 2010.

———. *Home Structure Fires*. Quincy, MA: National Fire Protection Association, Fire Analysis and Research Division, 2009.

———. *U.S. Experience with Smoke Alarms*. Quincy, MA: National Fire Protection Association, Fire Analysis and Research Division, 2004.

Ballesteros, M., M. Jackson, and M.W. Martin. Working towards the elimination of residential fire deaths: CDC's Smoke Alarm Installation and Fire Safety Education (SAIFE) Program. *J Burn Care Rehabil* (2005):26(5):434–9.

Flynn, J.D. *Characteristics of Home Fire Victims*. Quincy, MA: National Fire Protection Association, Fire Analysis and Research Division, 2008.

Harvey, P.A., M. Aitken, G.W. Ryan, et al. Strategies to increase smoke alarm use in high-risk households. *J Community Health* (2004):29(5):375–85.

Harvey, P.A., J.J. Sacks, G.W. Ryan, and P.F. Bender. Residential smoke alarms and fire escape plans. *Public Health Rep* (1998):113(5):459–64.

International Association for the Study of Insurance Economics. *World Fire Statistics: Information Bulletin of the World Fire Statistics*. Guelph, Ontario Canada: World Fire Statistics Center, Volume No. 25, October 2009.

Karter, M.J. *Fire Loss in the United States 2008*. Quincy, MA: National Fire Protection Association, Fire Analysis and Research Division, 2009.

National Center for Injury Prevention and Control. *Web-based Injury Statistics Query and Reporting System (WISQARS)* [Online]. (2006). Centers for Disease Control and Prevention (producer). Available at: http://www.cdc.gov/ncipc/wisqars. Accessed April 24, 2009.

National Fire Protection Association. *Harris Interactive Smoke Alarm Omnibus Question Report*. Quincy, MA; National Fire Protection Association, 2008.

Shaw, F.E., and C.P. Ogolla. Law, behavior, and injury prevention. In: Gielen, A.C., D.A. Sleet, and R.J. DiClemente, eds. *Injury and Violence Prevention: Behavioral Science Theories, Methods, and Applications*. San Francisco, CA: Jossey-Bass. 2006:442–66.

Thompson, N.J., M.B. Waterman, and D.A. Sleet. Using behavioral science to improve fire escape behaviors in response to a smoke alarm. *J Burn Care Rehabil* (2004):25(2):179–88.

U.S. Census Bureau. *American Housing Survey for the United States: 2007*. Available at: http://www.census.gov/hhes/www/housing/ahs/ahs07/ahs07.html. Accessed August 9, 2010.

Warda, L.J., and M.F. Ballesteros. Interventions to prevent residential fire injury. In: Doll, L.S., S.E. Bonzo, D.A. Sleet, J.A. Mercy, and E.N. Haas, eds. *Handbook of Injury and Violence Prevention*. New York: Springer, 2007:97–115.

Warda, L., M. Tenenbein, and M.E.K. Moffatt. House fire injury prevention update. Part I. A review of risk factors for fatal and non-fatal house fire injury. *Inj Prev* (1999):5:145–50.

Weatherization and Opportunities to Improve Health Conditions in Homes

Arnie Katz, MA Ed, and Ellen Tohn, MCP

Several factors are leading the nation toward what is likely to be a tidal wave of energy-related home improvement over the next decade. Billions of dollars will be spent during the next few years on projects referred to as "weatherization," "energy retrofit," and "energy efficiency improvements," in addition to broader remodeling or rehabilitation projects, with the goal of reducing the amount of energy used in our homes. The policy goals associated with these energy reductions are to decrease the energy expenditures of millions of Americans (many of them low income), reduce greenhouse gas emissions, and to potentially cut our dependence on foreign energy sources.

OVERVIEW OF WEATHERIZATION AND ENERGY EFFICIENCY ACTIVITIES

Home energy retrofits are typically done through one of several channels:

1. *Low-income Weatherization Assistance Program:* This is funded by the federal government; funds are dispersed to the states and then to local agencies in each community. The home assessments and work are done by the community agency, private contractors, or some combination of the two. The budget (nationally) for this program was approximately $200 million in 2009 and was increased to approximately $6 billion as part of the American Recovery and Reinvestment Act (stimulus package). As part of this change, the funds that can be expended in each home generally doubled from $3,000/housing unit to $6,000/housing unit. Several groups provide training and certification for those conducting auditing work (Building Performance Institute [BPI],

Residential Energy Services Network, Weatherization Assistance Program Technical Assistance Center). Training programs for weatherization energy efficiency improvements are also provided by BPI, Weatherization Assistance Program Technical Assistance Center, and others.

2. *Utility-subsidized energy improvement programs:* More and more states are requiring utilities to sponsor programs aimed at improving energy efficiency.

3. *Subsidized housing rehabilitation programs:* Typically funded by states, local governments, and the U.S. Department of Housing and Urban Development (HUD), these programs involve major work (often ≥ $20,000–$40,000) and are increasingly including advanced energy efficiency in their specifications.

4. *Private market activities:* Property owners increasingly are choosing to invest in making their homes or rental properties more energy efficient. The knowledge levels and competencies of the contractors doing this work run the gamut from highly knowledgeable and highly skilled to unskilled with little knowledge.

All of the energy efficiency approaches typically include certain basic procedures:

- air sealing (i.e., making the house/building tighter; reducing the infiltration [uncontrolled air flow coming into the home] of outside, unconditioned air and reducing the exfiltration [uncontrolled air flow leaving the home] of interior, conditioned air);
- sealing leaky ductwork, if there is ductwork in the house;
- adding additional attic insulation; and
- tuning up or replacing heating, ventilating, and air-conditioning equipment.

The percentage of residential buildings with ventilation systems is small, and of those the majority are relatively new (and not retrofit candidates) or they are homes in states with ventilation requirements. Homeowners may believe that their heating or air conditioning system includes ventilation when in fact it does not. For example, a survey of 100 new homes in North and South Carolina in 1994 turned up one house with a whole-house mechanical ventilation system (Katz 1997). In some parts of the country (e.g., Minnesota), ventilation has been code required, but just since the 1990s. Some high-performance home programs, such as Masco's *Environments for Living* (~150,000 homes) and Advanced Energy's *System Vision* program for affordable housing (~2,300 homes), have required whole-house ventilation, but they have existed for only approximately ten years, and these are not the homes that need energy retrofits. Similarly, homes built along the northern tier of the United States as part of an energy efficiency program often included a heat recovery ventilation system, but this is not a large percentage of homes, and, again, these are not the homes that are typically retrofit candidates.

A variety of other procedures are often included, such as wall or floor insulation, door and window repair, and installation of closed crawl-space systems. On the assumption that there is a national consensus about the importance of improving energy efficiency in houses while not making people sick or unintentionally causing moisture issues, this chapter describes both the risks to resident health and the opportunities to dramatically improve health conditions during widespread implementation of energy efficiency measures. An example of risk is that any time a house is tightened up (which includes tightening the duct system, unless it is totally inside the conditioned envelope of the home), the potential for concentrating contaminants and creating pressure differentials is increased. This can cause a variety of health, safety, durability, comfort, and energy use problems that did not exist previously. On the other hand, energy efficiency improvements done correctly can greatly minimize those risks and actually improve the health impacts of houses where problems previously existed.

FIRST, *DO NO HARM*

This phrase, taken from the medical world, expresses a concept that is absolutely central to understanding the relationships between making changes to houses and damaging or improving people's health. Any time someone enters a home to "fix" it, the home lies on a continuum from "toxic waste dump—get out immediately" to "benign—this house is more or less neutral in terms of health impacts" to "health-promoting—there are discernable aspects of this home that improve the health of the occupants" (Figure 10.1).

A goal of any home intervention should be to move the house toward the "health-promoting" end of the continuum. We should never do things to a house that change it in the direction of the "toxic" or harmful end of the spectrum. Although this seems obvious and self-evident, people can do things to houses that make them less healthy often in the name of "energy efficiency."

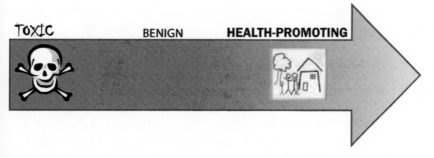

Source: *Courtesy of Advanced Energy.*

Figure 10.1—Health effects continuum.

Anyone who touches a home must understand the fundamental concept that "the house is a system." A house consists of various elements, such as the building shell; the heating, cooling, and ventilating equipment; and the air distribution ducts. Each of these elements interacts with each of the others: Change one, and you may inadvertently change another. Unless these interactions are understood and applied, there is substantial risk of exacerbating problems or even creating problems where none existed before the intervention.

Notably, those with fairly consistent access to trained, reasonably competent providers are only low-income families eligible for the Weatherization Assistance Program in states with strong weatherization training programs. Some utility programs include good training and quality services, but such are far from universal. For example, a few states, notably New York, California, and Wisconsin, have invested heavily in building an energy retrofit contractor infrastructure through the Home Performance with Energy Star program. Even in those states, however, there are not nearly as many quality contractors as will be required in the next few years, and there is no effective quality-control process in place.

Bringing in Contaminants

Homes that leak a lot of air have existing pathways that enable a variety of contaminants to "hitchhike" on air. Essentially, anything that is present in the outside air—pollen, dust, ozone, carbon monoxide, nitrogen oxides, sulfur oxides, particulates, and so forth—can enter the home. A leak in the return side of a forced-air system generally puts a house into a positive pressure state. If the leak is in an area where there are contaminants (e.g., a crawl space, attic, or garage), contaminants enter the living space. Leaky homes will be bringing in more outside air; whether the air is called "fresh" depends on where it is coming from. Because the source of all the air in the house is "outside," the presence of these contaminants in outside air will often lead to their presence inside. As the house is made tighter, the concentrations of contaminants can increase in the house if the removal rate is less than the entry rate.

Trapping Contaminants Created Inside in a Home

Similarly, some contaminants are generated by the house itself or by the heating or cooling equipment, furniture, pets, and people. Tightening up these houses can also increase contaminant concentrations by limiting dilution air and exfiltration pathways.

When tightening up a house, one should always consider the impact on both the intrusion and concentration of (1) moisture, (2) combustion by-products, (3) radon, (4) volatile organic compounds (VOCs), (5) environmental tobacco smoke, and (6) other particulates.

Moisture

Water, of course, is necessary to life. On the other hand, too much water in the wrong place can lead to a variety of human health problems. These include asthma, allergies, and other respiratory illnesses associated with dust mites, mold and other fungi, cockroaches, and rodents, all of which depend on moisture to grow and thrive (Institute of Medicine 2004). Similarly, the off-gassing of some VOCs, such as formaldehyde, can increase as relative humidity increases (Baughman and Arens 1996). Moisture management, therefore, must become part of the weatherization/ energy efficiency protocol to avoid creating health issues.

In cold climates, for instance, very leaky houses tend to be very dry in the winter. The infiltration of cold, dry air reduces the relative humidity inside the house. Tightening up the house can have the effect of increasing the relative humidity inside the house, because moist inside air is not being replaced with dry outside air. Although this may be desirable up to a point, the increase in relative humidity can increase the incidence of mold and other fungi, dust mites, insect pests, and other biological organisms that depend on the presence of moisture. The key is to find an acceptable balance. In addition, if a home is generally leaky and warm air generated in a bathroom or kitchen is naturally exhausting out cracks and holes that may be sealed during an energy efficiency improvement project, it is possible that moisture generated by combustion appliances or bathing, for example, can be trapped in the house, condense on surfaces, and lead to the growth of mold or other biological organisms.

In general, houses should not be made tighter if there are moisture issues present, unless the sources of the moisture problems are addressed. Roof leaks, plumbing leaks, interior condensation, and drainage problems can lead to negative health effects. If the house is made tighter while these problems persist, the health impacts may occur sooner and be worse. Fix the moisture problems first, then tighten the house.

Combustion By-Products

Many homes have appliances fueled by burning natural gas, propane, heating oil, kerosene, or wood. If these devices are located inside the heated space of the home, there is a risk that tightening the home will create pressure imbalances that can cause combustion by-products, including carbon monoxide, nitrogen oxides, water vapor, and soot, to be delivered into the home instead of outside via the chimney or flue. Exposure to high levels of carbon monoxide can result in death, and although the long-term effects of lower levels of exposure are not fully under-stood, the proximate effects include headaches, fatigue, and flu-like symptoms. Nitrogen oxides and small particles created by poorly operating systems can create respiratory issues. This is caused by negative pressure (pulling in air) in the zone of the home where the combustion is taking place. In practice, only a small amount of negative pressure can cause a furnace or water heater to backdraft combustion gasses into the home. In other words, furnaces, boilers, or water heaters that have been functioning adequately for years may cause serious health problems after the house is made tighter. Nitrogen oxides have also been found in kitchens as a result of poorly operating gas ranges.

The tighter the home is, the more likely it can hold pressure, and therefore the more likely it is to have a pressure-induced combustion issue. As we make the home tighter through weatherization and other energy retrofit activities, we must make sure that there are no atmospherically vented combustion devices inside the conditioned space or no substantial negative pressure created by the house (tested under worst-case conditions). Atmospherically vented furnaces and water heaters are the most common types in residential use. These types of combustion appliances rely on warm air rising to ensure that air used in the combustion process is exhausted outside. There is a space between the vent leading to the chimney and the top of the cabinet, open to the room that the device is in. This opening allows combustion gasses to be sucked out of the appliance and into the room.

In contrast, some newer models, called "direct vent," have no gap there, meaning the combustion gasses have no pathway into the house. In some houses, the conventional set-up is modified by installing a fan on the unit to bring in combustion air and make sure that the by-products are exhausted to the outside. Because the direct-vent and power-vented models are also more energy efficient, they are sometimes included in the energy retrofit.

Any home with combustion appliances, such as a gas or oil furnace, boiler, water heater, or oven, inside the conditioned envelope of the building (including basements) requires special attention. Homes with furnaces and water heaters can function well until the home is weatherized, at which point appliances begin to back draft and dump combustion gasses, such as carbon monoxide, nitrogen oxides, and water vapor, into the house.

There are only three acceptable approaches to this issue:

1. Remove all atmospherically vented (standard) equipment from the house (including the basement) and replace it with either direct-vent (sealed combustion or power-vented) equipment or non-combustion equipment (e.g., electric heat pumps).

2. Move the equipment outside of the conditioned envelope or build a tight enclosure around the equipment, connected to the outside.

3. Test the house using the combustion safety protocol of the BPI (http://www.bpi. org/documents/Gold_Sheet.pdf). Have the test performed by a qualified technician

to establish that, at least on the day of the testing, there is no backdrafting or spillage of combustion by-products into the living space.

Houses with combustion equipment should not be made tighter without implementing one of the strategies listed. Under no circumstances should houses be made tighter if there are unvented space heaters present. There are no safe applications of these devices in residential structures. Reducing outside air infiltration by making a house tighter in the presence of an unvented combustion device is likely to make an already unsafe condition even worse. For similar reasons, gas ovens and ranges should always have a range hood vented to the outside.

Radon

Radon is a cancer-causing natural radioactive gas that cannot be seen or smelled. According to the Environmental Protection Agency (EPA), radon is the leading cause of lung cancer among nonsmokers and the second leading cause of lung cancer in America. Exposure to radon claims approximately 20,000 lives annually (EPA 2003).

All houses should be tested both before and after any air-sealing project to ensure that the radon level does not exceed EPA or World Health Organization (WHO) thresholds. The EPA action level is 4 picocuries (pCi) per liter, and the World Health Organization action level is 2.7 pCi. Short-term radon test kits can measure radon in a 48-hour period; these radon tests are relatively low cost and readily available. There are documented examples of homes that tested below the threshold level before weatherization but tested above the threshold level after being tightened up (Dastur et al. 2009). If a home tests above the action-level threshold before work begins, radon mitigation should be included in the scope of work. In most cases, radon mitigation is outside of the budget of weatherization work, but at a minimum weatherization work in homes with radon levels exceeding the EPA threshold should not increase radon exposures and homeowners/occupants should be informed of the radon risks. In some cases, including the basics of a passive radon mitigation system in the weatherization/energy efficiency work makes sense even if the pre-test does not indicate radon at or above the action level. It may be less costly to include radon mitigation at this time instead of waiting until after weatherization is done, particularly if weatherization involves repairs to the basement or crawl space. This would be particularly appropriate in buildings with no slab, that is, dirt-floor crawl spaces or basements. This is common in the Southeast, parts of the Mid-Atlantic region, the Northwest, and parts of the Midwest.

Volatile Organic Compounds

Sources of VOCs in houses include cleaning products; paints, varnishes, and other finishes being used or stored in the house; gasoline in lawn mowers and other equipment, stored in attached garages, basements, or other attached spaces; off-gassing from carpeting, dry cleaning, furniture, and cabinets; landscape/garden products, such as pesticides and fertilizers; household pesticides; hairsprays and other cosmetics; various "air-freshening" products; candles and incense; and many others.

The number and variety of VOC sources in homes make generalizations difficult. At a minimum, anyone contemplating making a home tighter should do a basic assessment of potential VOC contamination. If there are indications of substantial VOC exposures in the home (visual observation of potential VOC sources, e.g., pesticides, fertilizers, gasoline, kerosene, cleaning agents; odors; occupant reports of respiratory illness), these factors should be taken into account when developing an air-sealing strategy. Such a strategy should include the following:

- occupant education about the possible relationships between VOC sources in the home and health impacts on the occupants; and

- exploration of possible ways to isolate large VOC sources from the living space. Examples include air-sealing between the living space and an attached garage or using an exhaust fan to depressurize the garage relative to the house, guaranteeing that any air flow between them will go from the house to the garage and not from the garage to the house. This strategy can also be used in a closet or even a cabinet.

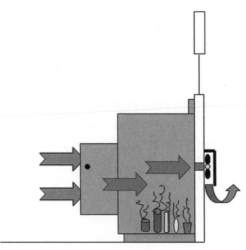

Source: Courtesy of Advanced Energy.

Figure 10.2 — Cabinet exhaust.

Figure 10.2 shows an under-counter cabinet storing several containers giving off VOCs. An exhaust fan has been installed at the rear of the cabinet, with the switch connected to the cabinet door. When the door is opened, the fan comes on, pulling the air (and the VOCs) out of the house instead of allowing them to enter the living space. The cabinet must be well sealed for this to be effective.

Environmental Tobacco Smoke

Any effort to tighten a home will invariably trap tobacco smoke that is created in a house. The best response to this situation is to encourage residents to smoke outside, explaining that once the contractor has tightened up the home for energy savings, it will be less leaky and tobacco smoke will be more likely to stay in the home.

RISK AND BEST PRACTICES WHEN DISTURBING OR DECONSTRUCTING EXISTING HOUSING COMPONENTS

Lead

As discussed in Chapter 2, lead-based paint was banned in 1978 by the Consumer Product Safety Commission. By the mid-1950s, many paint manufacturers had begun reducing the lead content in paint. Approximately 69% of homes built before 1960 and approximately 87% built before 1940 have lead-based paint (National Center for Healthy Housing 2009; U.S. Environment Protection Agency 1995). Many energy efficiency and weatherization jobs may not create problems with lead because the work does not cut, sand, demolish, or otherwise disturb old painted surfaces that are likely to have lead-based paint. However, at least one study has shown that even the blower door test to assess the tightness of a home can generate lead dust. Some common weatherization and energy efficiency projects do disturb paint, which, if it contains lead, can produce lead dust at levels that can exceed the EPA standards. For example, replacing windows and cutting holes in walls or ceilings to install insulation have been shown to produce harmful levels of lead dust in homes that have lead-based paint (National Center for Healthy Housing 2007). One task that can disturb paint but did not result in elevated dust lead loadings in field testing was scraping doors to install weather-stripping.

The EPA and HUD have numerous documents that describe safe practices for work that may disturb lead-based paint (http://www.hud.gov/offices/cpd/affordable housing/training/web/leadsafe/keyrequirements/safepractices.cfm; http://www.epa.gov/lead/pubs/contractor_brochure.pdf). In general, such practices seek to:

- contain and control the creation or spread of lead paint chips and dust by selecting tools and practices that minimize the creation of lead dust/chips and using plastic sheeting and other containment measures to limit the spread of any such dust outside the work area;
- clean up lead dust using a combination of high-efficiency particulate air (HEPA) or high-efficiency vacuums followed by a comprehensive wet clean-up where dirty and rinse water are kept separate; and
- perform post-cleanup dust testing, in some cases, to ensure that elevated dust lead loadings do not persist.

The EPA Renovation, Repair, and Painting rule applies to all housing built before 1978, where the work will disturb more than 6 square feet in the interior or 20 square feet on the exterior of the house (40 CFR 745.86). This exemption for small jobs does not apply to the following: window replacement; demolition of painted surface areas; use of open-flame burning or torching; use of machines to remove paint through high-speed operation without HEPA exhaust control; or operation of a heat gun at temperatures of 1,100°F or greater. Under the rule, beginning in April 2010, contractors performing renovation, repair, and painting projects that disturb lead-based paint in homes, child care facilities, and schools built before 1978 must be certified and must follow specific work practices to prevent lead contamination (see http://www.epa.gov).

Asbestos

Asbestos can be found in homes most frequently in piping insulation, boiler insulation, floor tiles, siding, and roof tiles. Energy efficiency work that entails upgrading or replacing heating and cooling systems, cutting holes in exterior siding to blow in insulation, or repairing roofs before installation of air sealing or attic insulation may disturb asbestos-containing components. Work that makes asbestos fibers inhalable can increase risks for lung cancer, mesothelioma (a cancer of the lining of the chest and abdominal cavity), and asbestosis (when lungs become scarred with fibrous tissue).

The EPA's recommendations related to asbestos are to avoid disturbing the material when at all possible. If the insulation or shingles are disturbed during repair or replacement projects, follow state regulations related to asbestos removal.

Insulation

Disturbing old insulation can create risks of exposure to both occupants and workers. Primary exposure risks are to:
1. airborne fiberglass fibers;
2. airborne mineral wool fibers;

3. airborne cellulose fibers; and

4. accumulated dust and other contaminants, such as dead insects and rodents, droppings of various animals, including bats, squirrels, snakes, rodents, and so forth.

Workers should always wear respirators. Old insulation should be bagged in place before being carried through the house. When possible, leave it in place and add new insulation to it.

Do Not Expose Occupants to Potentially Hazardous or Harmful Materials

Work to improve energy efficiency may also involve using products. Efforts should be taken to ensure that any new products introduced into a home do not expose residents to potentially harmful materials.

INSULATION

Some insulation products can cause allergic or other respiratory problems. Minimize exposures for occupants by keeping materials bagged when carried through the living space whenever possible and cleaning up any dropped or spilled material. Some insulation products may contain formaldehyde, which may off-gas over time. Other products contain various binders and fire retardants, which sometimes lead to allergic reactions in sensitive individuals. Workers installing spray foams should take special care to use the appropriate protective equipment and procedures to avoid exposures to chemicals that can result in respiratory problems, skin irritation, and other health concerns.

Combustion Appliances

When installing new combustion appliances (e.g., water heaters, furnaces, or boilers) inside the conditioned space, it is always preferable to install direct-vent (sealed combustion or power-vented) units. A direct-vent unit is one that brings outside air for combustion directly into the burner, which is connected directly to the outside by a vent pipe that cannot allow combustion gasses to escape into the building. Often, these are vented through the wall with a "pipe within a pipe" configuration so that one hole in the wall handles both the incoming air and the exhaust gasses. If that is not feasible, isolate the appliance from the conditioned space (through air-sealing and insulation), being sure to supply adequate combustion and dilution air per code. As an alternative, certify that the installation is not backdrafting—and will not backdraft—according to the BPI Combustion Safety Protocol.

Paint

Use low-VOC paint. Some third-party organizations, such as Greenseal and the Canadian Ecologo program, certify paints for low VOCs (e.g., http://www.greenseal. org; http://www.terrachoice-certified.com). It is also useful to consider whether the use of paint or other finishes is actually necessary. Although most people prefer the finished look, this is primarily an aesthetic rather than a durability decision. Homeowners who like the look of unfinished wood present an opportunity to reduce exposures to VOCs.

Caulk

Some caulks may contain formaldehyde. Although the potential exposures to occupants are not well documented, a precautionary approach would be to seek out caulks that do not contain formaldehyde.

OPPORTUNITIES TO IMPROVE HEALTH FOR RESIDENTS

Beyond avoiding unintended health problems during energy efficiency work, the potential exists to improve health conditions in homes. Weatherization and other energy retrofits typically entail multiple visits characterized by an audit or assessment to diagnose issues and one or more visits by contractors to complete the work. This sequencing offers opportunities to both identify housing-related health concerns to address and to incorporate health-driven specifications into the job. Some of the improvements will be useful to all residents, regardless of age or susceptibility to an illness, whereas others are more appropriate for particular individuals or situations (e.g., reducing asthma triggers for an asthmatic person and installing improved lighting or grab bars for the elderly to minimize trip and fall hazards). Common opportunities for improvements are described next.

Keep It Dry

Common repairs that can enhance health conditions when undertaking energy efficiency or weatherization work include the following:
- repair roof to ensure that attic insulation stays dry;
- repair door and window flashing when such components are being replaced to minimize future problems;
- repair gutters, downspouts, and grading to more effectively manage rainwater;
- install water leak detection alarms or drains near water heaters, which when they fail can create extreme moisture problems if not detected early;

- repair plumbing leaks;
- install high-quality bathroom exhaust fan (discussed later); and
- install high-quality kitchen exhaust hood (discussed later).

Crawl spaces are often damp and dank places, yet air is sometimes pulled from these locations to ventilate homes or the homes inadvertently allow the movement of air from crawl spaces into the occupied space. If there are signs of water in the crawl space (puddles, past staining), the source(s) should be identified (e.g., inadequate drainage, improper site grading, blocked or broken gutters/downspouts, inadequate foundation damp-proofing, plumbing leaks) and repaired before other work in the crawl space. Typically, a sealed vapor retarder, such as a polyethylene sheet at least 6 millimeters thick, should be installed covering 100% of the ground and up the walls to at least 12 inches above the exterior grade, being careful to leave a 2–3-inch termite view strip in those areas subject to subterranean termites. In much of the United States, unvented crawl spaces (particularly in the Southeast and Northwest) have been shown to be drier than vented crawl spaces. For specific details and research reports, refer to http://www.crawlspaces.org and http://www.buildingscience.com/documents/insights/bsi-009-new-light-in-crawlspaces.

Keep It Ventilated

Because making a house more airtight increases the probabilities of moisture problems, combustion gas problems, and other contaminant problems, implementing a ventilation strategy can substantially reduce the likelihood of creating those problems. Implementing appropriate ventilation strategies can actually improve the quality of the interior environment, making a positive contribution to the health of the people in the house.

Local or spot ventilation can remove moisture or other contaminants from a specific area of the building. Typically, this consists of installing exhaust fans in bathrooms (to remove moisture and odors), kitchens (to remove moisture, odors, and combustion gas by-products), and home workshops (to remove fumes from solvents and other VOCs). Sometimes, it is advisable to install a local exhaust fan in attached garages or closets/cabinets holding VOCs, such as paints, stains, pesticides, gasoline, and fertilizer.

All exhaust fans should be tested after installation to ensure that the specifications described next are met. They should always be ducted through the exterior skin of the building to the outside and fitted with a proper termination. "Outside" does not include in attic, crawl space, or basement. Venting to these spaces can actually increase moisture or contaminant issues by sending warm, humid air or contaminant-laden air to other spots in the home. Vinyl flex duct or other "flimsy" materials should not be used, as they tend not to hold up well over time.

Ventilation ducts going through unconditioned space (e.g., attics) should be insulated to avoid condensation.

Bathrooms: Install a quiet (<1 sone) fan that moves at least 50 cubic feet per minute out of the bathroom. A "sone" is a unit of perceived loudness. The best practice standards for ventilation specified in American Society of Heating, Refrigerating and Air-Conditioning Engineers (ASHRAE) 62.2 require a fan with a maximum of 1.0 sone if operating continuously and a maximum of 3 sones if operating intermittently (ASHRAE 2010).

Kitchen: ASHRAE 62.2 also recommends installing a quiet fan (<3 sones) over a range that moves at least 100 cubic feet per minute out of the kitchen.

Whole-house ventilation: Currently, the best guidance on ventilation in houses is ASHRAE 62.2. The standard clarifies its intent related to whole-house ventilation as follows: "Whole-house ventilation is intended to dilute the unavoidable contaminant emissions from people, from materials, and from background processes" (ASHRAE 2010). The current ASHRAE standard provides guidance to select a system for a given house. These systems may be exhaust only, supply only, or exhaust and supply.

Exhaust only: At the lower-cost end are systems that use exhaust fans (bathroom fans or separate, dedicated exhaust fans) running continuously at low speed. Be sure to install a fan that is rated for continuous operation, because most bath fans are not. The primary drawback of this approach is that as inside air is exhausted, outside air will be drawn into the house through random cracks and holes. This could mean that the outside air is coming in through the moldy crawl-space or dusty attic, or from next to the termiticide-saturated foundation. In other words, outside air is not the same as "fresh" air.

Supply only: Another relatively low-cost approach is to bring outside air into the return-air side of the heating/cooling system. The intake should be located in as "clean" an area as possible, and the air should be filtered before being circulated throughout the house. The outside air is mixed with the air in the house and heated or cooled before being circulated throughout the house.

Combination exhaust and supply: Typically, these systems are considerably more expensive, but they have the advantage of being much more energy efficient. In northern climates, a heat recovery ventilator captures much of the heat from the air being exhausted and transfers that heat to the outside air coming in. In southern climates, an energy recovery ventilator removes much of the moisture from the incoming air and transfers it to the air being exhausted. Both heat and energy recovery ventilators will bring in outside air with little energy penalty. In addition, these systems balance the amount of air coming in and going out, so they do not create any pressure imbalance (positive or negative) in the house.

It is crucial, however, that some form of ventilation be installed in houses, even if there is an energy penalty. Energy efficiency is extremely important for a number of reasons, but should never be achieved at the expense of the health of families in their houses.

Keep It Pest Free

Pest droppings in homes can be triggers for asthma and result in increased use of pesticides. Pests generally enter homes and buildings through holes and cracks, precisely the types of situations that energy efficiency contractors can identify. These entryways can be sealed with modest adjustments in diagnostics procedures and use of materials. Now in addition to stopping the flow of air, contractors will work to eliminate entryways that pests use to come inside. This in turn means that residents no longer need pesticides to deal with pest problems. The end result is reduced toxins in the home.

The three most common pests with known or likely linkages to asthma triggers or respiratory concerns are mice, rats, and cockroaches (Institute of Medicine 2000). Rats, like other rodents, may also carry diseases. Data from the American Housing Survey indicate that approximately 1% of homes have rats and 6% of homes report mice issues (U.S. Census Bureau 2006). The American Housing Survey did not include questions related to cockroaches. Rodents typically enter near foundations and can enter surprisingly small holes. For example, a mouse can squeeze through a hole the size of a dime, whereas a rat needs a larger hole. Roaches need even less space. A good resource on excluding pests from your home is "How to Control Pests Safely" (available at http://www.nyc.gov/html/doh/downloads/pdf/pest/pest-bro-healthy-home.pdf).

Seal Points of Entry

Where to look: During the audit or initial visit, in addition to looking or testing for air leakage using a blower door, look for evidence of pests droppings or ask residents where they have pest problems. In some cases it may be useful to put out cockroach or mice traps to document the pest infestation locations to focus responses.

How to seal holes for rodents: Although most air-sealing crews are familiar with caulk guns and expanding foam, these materials will not last in the long run against a determined rodent or squirrel. It is best to add a corrosion-proof metal (e.g., copper mesh) that the mice and rats cannot chew through to the sealing process. Some combination of metal and low-VOC caulking or other sealant usually will do the job. Sealing from the outside is more effective at preventing pest entry than sealing from the inside. Installing a hardware cloth (1/4-inch wire mesh) on the outside of the foundation can also help prevent rodent entry.

How to keep cockroaches outside: Once the location of the roach problem is identified, it is always useful to walk outside and determine whether there may be a trash problem that could be contributing to the infestation. To seal up cracks and holes that let cockroaches into homes, look for the holes/cracks inside and outside. Seal holes and cracks with caulk, and if possible, use a licensed pesticide applicator to apply boric acid inside the hole/crack before sealing it up. Explain to the resident that good housekeeping, in conjunction with baits and gels, will also help address the problem.

Where to Seal

Rodents: Look along the foundation inside the home and outside. Examine penetrations to the exterior walls or signs of burrowing.

Roaches: Look inside for pest droppings and nearby cracks or holes. Common problem areas are kitchens and other areas with food.

Keep It Contaminant Free

COMBUSTION

- All combustion appliances (water heaters, furnaces, boilers, heaters, fireplaces) installed inside the conditioned space should be direct-vent (sealed combustion or power-vented) or certified combustion safe according to the BPI combustion safety protocol.
- All combustion ranges and ovens should be checked for efficient, safe operation and accompanied by an exhaust hood ducted to the outside.
- Attached garages: To the extent possible, all holes between the living space and the garage should be sealed. In addition, use pressure-control strategies to make sure that any flow between the house and the garage is moving the air from the house to the garage and not from the garage to the house. This can be accomplished by pressurizing the house with reference to the garage by bringing outside air into the house or by installing an exhaust fan in the garage, thereby creating a lower pressure in the garage.

LEAD

EPA regulations now require the use of lead-safe practices for work that disturbs more than 2 feet inside and 20 feet on the exterior in homes built before 1978. These requirements are described earlier in this chapter.

In addition to doing no harm when it comes to lead, lead hazards can be reduced during energy upgrades. When working on a home built before 1978, especially those built before 1960, any renovation job including energy efficiency work is an opportunity to repair non-intact paint or replace building components that have older flaking, peeling paint or older paint that rubs and creates dust.

Windows: Although window replacement is not standard in most weatherization jobs or energy efficiency jobs because of the lengthier payback relative to other energy efficiency measures, this type of replacement can remove a building component that often is the source of lead paint chips and dust found on window sills.

Doors: Similarly, older doors with peeling paint that may not fit snugly may be an opportunity to replace a component containing leaded paint with a lead-free door that is weather-stripped to fit snugly and reduce air leakage.

Other peeling, flaking paint: Homes with visible peeling paint, particularly on the inside or front porch, have a substantially increased risk of containing higher lead dust loadings inside. Weatherization and energy efficiency work may be an opportunity to stabilize the paint using lead-safe work practice and clean up any lead dust that may have been inside the living space as part of the paint repair cleanup.

Entryway walk-off systems: Another effective and relatively low-cost measure to minimize the spread of lead dust inside from exterior sources is to install entryway walk-off systems. Approximately two-thirds of the dust and debris in our homes is tracked inside from outdoors. Walk-off systems that have an exterior mat or grate combined with an interior mat can help remove contaminants brought inside on shoes. For example, the U.S. Green Building Council's *LEED for Homes* standard, which applies to homes with fewer than four stories, includes a green criterion for optional points to minimize track in of contaminants by installation of a walk-off mat that is at least 4 feet long or provision of permanent storage for shoes near entryways to encourage shoe removal (U.S. Green Building Council 2007).

RADON

Testing before work begins: Because many jobs may change the flow of air into and out of the building, it is useful to document radon levels before work begins. Such testing is strongly recommended for single-family homes in high-risk radon areas where the living spaces may be in close contact with the crawl spaces or basement. The EPA maintains a web listing of high-risk radon areas, and some states have more specific information (http://www.epa.gov/radon). For more information about testing procedures, go to http://www.epa.gov/radon. A short-term test can be performed in 48 hours. Some states require radon measurement testers to follow a specific testing protocol. If the contractor or auditor performs the test, carefully follow the testing protocol for your area or EPA's Radon Testing Checklist. When hiring a contractor to test the residence, it is important to select a qualified individual or company. Check with your state radon office, which can be found online at http://www.epa.gov/iaq/whereyoulive.html, for more information.

If the results exceed or are very close to 4 pCi/L, care should be taken to not increase the pull of radon gas into the home or trap radon that may already be entering the home. Air sealing and other energy efficiency measures that reduce air leakage out of a home could contain more radon gas in a home. Radon levels in excess of 4 pCi/L can be addressed through a variety of measures, some of which could be added to an energy efficiency job. The EPA (1993) has produced a useful guide to radon-resistant construction in existing homes.

Post-work testing: If the initial reading exceeded the EPA Action Level of 4 pCi/L, radon testing after the job is done is recommended to ensure that the energy efficiency work did not inadvertently increase radon levels. Such post-work testing can protect contractors in all settings to document that the efficiency work did not increase radon exposures for occupants.

Radon remediation: The EPA has produced several documents that detail radon-resistant construction in both new and existing homes and buildings. The EPA estimates that the costs of radon-resistant construction range from $800 to $2,500 per home. Typical radon-control systems involve sealing the foundation to minimize movement of radon gas through the slab into the building and installing systems to trap the gas under the slab and exhaust it out of the home through a series of pipes that atmospherically vent the gas or use a fan to suck the gas out.

VOLATILE ORGANIC COMPOUNDS

For some individuals, exposures to VOCs commonly found in homes in cleaning, painting, varnishing, pest control, air freshener, and personal care products can result in eye, nose, and throat irritation; headaches, loss of coordination, and nausea; and damage to the liver, kidneys, and central nervous system (EPA 2009a). During energy efficiency work, consulting with the homeowner or tenant presents opportunities to:

- remove products containing VOCs that are not needed in the home (e.g., old cleaning products, paint, varnishes);
- relocate storage of VOC-containing products outside key living spaces to the garage, basement, or other areas and install an exhaust fan in the storage area to maintain it at a negative pressure with reference to the living space; and
- create an "off-gassing closet" with an exhaust fan that can be used to reduce off-gassing from items brought into the home, such as freshly dry-cleaned clothing. At least one large national home builder is currently installing these as a standard feature in its homes. Similarly, it is useful to review the VOC content of insulation by examining the Material Safety Data Sheet.

PESTICIDES

The majority of Americans store pesticides in their homes. Keeping these products outside of the reach of children is critical to minimize the risk of poisoning or contamination of food or cooking equipment if pesticides are stored in a kitchen. Energy work offers an opportunity to advise homeowners and tenants on proper storage of pesticides and how to read labels to avoid unintended health issues from misuse or overuse.

Education also may help owners understand the role of integrated pest management techniques in addressing pest issues. Integrated pest management strategies address pest infestations through observation of pests to ensure that the treatment targets the problem; exclusion of pests by sealing holes and cracks to the outside; proper housekeeping and food storage to minimize situations that attract pests; and selected use of low-toxicity pesticides.

OTHER CONTAMINANTS

Candles: The burning of candles inside the home can be a significant source of soot and other particulate (Vigil 1998). Soot deposits (e.g., on ceilings, walls, refrigerators, computers, and carpets) may be an indicator of candle use, although other sources may be responsible. Candle use is sometimes associated with annoying odors that people are trying to cover up. This is an opportunity to help the occupants identify and eliminate the source of the odors.

Air fresheners: Similarly, the use of air fresheners suggests odors or other conditions in the home that may be unhealthy. Identifying the sources of the odors and eliminating them, rather than attempting to mask them, is generally preferable.

Keep It Clean

Install walk-off systems: Install an outside mat or grate in combination with an interior mat. This strategy is relatively low cost and helps to reduce the track in of contaminants, including pesticides, lead, other metals, and allergens.

Upgrade air filtration: On forced-air heating, cooling, or ventilation systems that filter air, ensure the air filter has at least a Minimum Efficiency Reporting Value (MERV) of 8 if the system can handle the upgraded filtration level. This needs to be determined by a qualified technician. A MERV 10 is preferable if consistent with system operations and warranties (U.S. Green Building Council 2008). The higher the MERV rating, the better the filter is at collecting particles of various sizes and keeping them out of the air. However, installing a better filter can sometimes put strain on the motor and lead to premature failure of the system. Most filters on heating and air conditioning systems protect the equipment and have nothing to do with improving the air quality in the home. Although it is often possible to install a filter that will contribute to better air quality, it is always advisable to make sure the system will not be harmed.

Work with residents to reduce and properly store cleaning products: Many homes contain a host of relatively toxic cleaning products, many of which are used infrequently. These products also may be stored under the kitchen cabinet or in other locations that are easily accessible to children. Weatherization and energy efficiency work typically involves emptying kitchen sink cabinets to ensure that plumbing penetrations are property sealed. When these products are removed, it is a good opportunity to work with the homeowner or resident to ask:

- Do you still use this product?
- Is there a less toxic alternative that could be used? Consider providing the following green cleaning recipe (Figure 10.3) or a list of green products.
- If you do not use the product, where can you safely dispose of it?
- What pesticides are under the sink and are they safe?

Foggers are not a good choice (Kass et al. 2009) because they are limited in their effectiveness in dealing with cockroaches and, in some cases, have caused explosions. EPA guidance explains that because the aerosol propellants in these foggers typically are flammable, improper use may cause a fire or explosion. In addition to this hazard, failure to vacate premises during fogging or reentering without airing out may result in illness (EPA 2009b).

Keep It Safe

Several opportunities exist to improve the safety in a home that is undergoing weatherization or energy efficiency.

Install smoke alarms: Such alarms often are required by code. The alarms ideally should be hard wired with battery back-up (see Chapter 9).

1 quart warm water
1 teaspoon liquid soap
1 teaspoon borax
½ cup undiluted white vinegar

Do not use on marmoleum

Figure 10.3—All purpose green cleaner.

Install carbon monoxide alarms: Some states require such alarms. It is best to use alarms with a digital read-out and a button that allows the user to see the peak level (a peak level button).

Minimize trip and fall hazards: These actions are particularly helpful for older residents. Useful measures include installation of grab bars in showers, bath, and bathrooms near toilets; installation of hand rails on stairs; improved lighting and night lights near bathrooms, improved exterior lighting; and, for homes with young children, installation of stair gates at the top and bottom of stairs to prevent toddlers from falling.

Minimize poisoning risk: Install childproof cabinet locks for cabinets that may hold pesticides, chemicals, or other products that could cause poisonings.

Install childproof outlet covers or plugs: In some homes, there may be some energy savings associated with this, but the big advantage is helping prevent children from sticking things into outlets.

KEEP IT MAINTAINED

Spot ventilation: Check both the intakes and terminations of all exhaust fans, including the dryer. These are often clogged with dust, lint, or dead pests. If this is the case, educate the occupants about the importance of periodically cleaning these areas so the exhaust fans can work. In addition, regular cleaning of the dryer exhaust duct will reduce the chance of house fires and improve the efficiency of the dryer.

Filtration change: Similarly, check the furnace and air conditioner filters. If they are clogged, educate the occupants about the importance of periodically changing the filter so that the system will last longer and provide greater comfort for less money.

CONCLUSION

As a guide for contractors and program coordinators, Table 10.1 presents healthy housing activities that often are associated with energy upgrades, grouped into three categories: (1) precautions to avoid increasing health risks for occupants ("Do No Harm"), (2) relatively low-cost actions to improve occupant health ("Low-Cost Health Improvements"), and (3) higher-cost actions that may be appropriate on a given job and may improve occupant health ("Additional Health Improvement Opportunities"). During the next decade, we will witness an unprecedented effort to improve the energy efficiency of all buildings in America, including our homes. Careful attention to detail and awareness of opportunities to improve

TABLE 10.1 — ACTIONS FOR ENERGY EFFICIENCY PLUS HEALTH

Do No Harm	Low-Cost Health Improvements	Additional Health Improvement Opportunities
Keep It Dry		
• Do not insulate or air seal attic until vented appliances to attic are exhausted outside (e.g., bath fan, dryer exhaust).	• Add pan flashing to all window replacements.	• Eliminate standing water problems. • Repair interior and exterior water leaks and poorly managed rainwater.
Keep It Ventilated		
• Do not tighten house if unvented combustion appliances are present or atmospherically vented combustion appliances are in the conditioned space.	• Ensure that all clothes dryers exhaust to the outside. • All newly installed heating/cooling or hot water combustion equipment is direct or power vented.	• Install direct or power-vented equipment or certify (after energy work is complete) that negative pressures > 3 Pa cannot be created in the combustion appliance zones.
	• Replace or install exterior vented bath fans meeting ASHRAE 62.2. • Existing or newly installed central forced-air HVAC system(s) have minimum MERV 8 filter, no filter bypass, and no ozone generators.	• Retrofit/commission to meet ASHRAE standard 62.2 for whole house and kitchen exterior exhausting fan.
Avoid Contaminants		
• Test for radon before and after work to ensure work does not trap radon.	• Certified low-VOC or no-VOC interior paints and finishes used.	• Repair deteriorated paint with lead-safe work practices.
• Use lead-safe practices (i.e., EPA's renovation and remodeling rule).	• Recommend no smoking indoors.	• Mitigate radon to ASTM 2121 if > 4 pC/L.
• Do not disturb vermiculite or asbestos.		• New pressed wood products, specify compliance with California Air Resources Board's low-formaldehyde standards (e.g., plywood, OSB, MDF, cabinetry).
		• Air seal attached garages to prevent entry of volatile substances and carbon monoxide into living areas.
		• Carpet, adhesives, and cushions qualify for CRI Green Label Plus or Green Label testing program.

TABLE 10.1—ACTIONS FOR ENERGY EFFICIENCY PLUS HEALTH (CONTINUED)

Do No Harm	Low-Cost Health Improvements	Additional Health Improvement Opportunities
Keep It Safe		
	• Install smoke and carbon monoxide alarms. • Educate residents about fire safety.	• Install grab bars in showers, bathtubs, and near toilets. • Install hand rails on stairs, and improve lighting and night lights near bathrooms. • For homes with young children, install stair gates at the top and bottom of stairs. • Install childproof cabinet locks for cabinets that may hold pesticides, chemicals, or other products.
Keep It Clean		
	• Install walk-off mats or grates.	• Remove and replace worn carpets with resilient flooring.
	• Provide sealable garbage cans.	• Provide mattress/bed covers for families with breathing problems; provide a vacuum cleaner and containers to keep materials off the ground.
Keep It Pest Free		
	• Patch exterior holes using pest-resistant materials (e.g., copper mesh or caulk). Apply boric acid or gels in holes for roach issues.	• Install airtight sump covers.
Maintain the Home		
	• Educate residents about preventing indoor environmental problems.	

ASHRAE = American Society of Heating, Refrigerating, and Air-Conditioning Engineers; ASTM = American Society for Testing and Materials; CRI = Carpet and Rug Institute; EPA = Environmental Protection Agency; HVAC = heating, ventilating, and air-conditioning; MDF = medium-density fiberboard; MERV = Minimum Efficiency Reporting Value; OSB = oriented strand board; VOC = volatile organic compound. Courtesy of Tohn Environmental Strategies and the National Center for Healthy Housing.

health conditions for homeowners and renters will ensure that our national commitment to energy conservation and efficiency also reaps health benefits. There are tremendous opportunities to embed health concerns and awareness into training, protocols, and delivery mechanism for government- and utility-funded work. The challenge confronting health professionals is to build these bridges and to ensure that energy efficiency work is also healthy.

REFERENCES

American Society of Heating, Refrigerating, and Air-Conditioning Engineers. *Standard 62.2 Ventilation and Acceptable Indoor Air Quality in Low Rise Residential Buildings* (2010).

Baughman, A.V., and E.A. Arens. Indoor humidity and human health—Part I: Literature review of health effects of humidity-influenced indoor pollutants. *ASHRAE Transactions: Research* (1996):193–211.

Dastur, C., M. Mancer, B. Hannas, and D. Novosel. *Closed Crawlspace Performance: Proof of Concept in the Production Builder Marketplace.* Alexandria, VA: National Center for Energy Management and Building Technology; 2009: http://www.advancedenergy.org/buildings/knowledge_library/crawl_spaces/pdfs/NCEMBT%20Report.pdf. Accessed July 12, 2010.

Institute of Medicine. *Clearing the Air: Asthma and Indoor Air Exposures.* Washington, DC: National Academies Press, 2000.

——. *Damp Indoor Spaces and Health.* Washington, DC: National Academies Press, 2004.

Kass, D., W. McKelvey, E. Carlton, et al. Effectiveness of an integrated pest management intervention in controlling cockroaches, mice, and allergens in New York City public housing. *Environ Health Perspect* (2009):1219–25.

Katz, A. What's being built out there. *Home Energy Magazine* (1997):29–34.

National Center for Healthy Housing. *The Analysis of Lead-Safe Weatherization Practices and the Presence of Lead in Weatherized Homes* (2007). Available at: http://www.nchh.org/Research/Archived-Research-Projects/Weatherization-and-Lead-Safety.aspx. Accessed February 11, 2010.

——. *National Healthy Homes Training Center Curriculum* (2009). Available at: http://www.healthyhomestraining.org/Curriculum/index.htm. Accessed February 11, 2009.

U.S. Census Bureau. *American Housing Survey for the United States: 2005.* Washington, DC: U.S. Government Printing Office, 2006. Available at: http://www.census.gov/hhes/www/housing/ahs/ahs05/ahs05.html. Accessed July 12, 2010.

U.S. Environmental Protection Agency. *An Introduction to Indoor Air Quality* (2009a). Available at: http://www.epa.gov/iaq/ia-intro.html. Accessed February 11, 2010.

——. *Assessment of Risks from Radon in Homes* (2003). Washington, DC. Available at: http://www.epa.gov/radon/pdfs/402-r-03-003.pdf. Accessed July 12, 2010.

——. *Radon Reduction Techniques for Existing Detached Houses: Technical Guidance for Active Soil Depressurization Systems, 3rd ed.* (1993). (EPA 625/R-93-011).

——. *Report on the National Survey of Lead-Based Paint in Housing: Base Report* (1995). Available at: http://www.epa.gov/lead/pubs/r95-003.pdf. Accessed July 12, 2010.

——. *Safety Precautions for Total Release Foggers* (2009b). Available at: http://www.epa.gov/opp00001/factsheets/fogger.htm. Accessed February 11, 2010.

U.S. Green Building Council. *LEED for Homes.* Washington, DC: U.S. Green Building Council, 2007.

——. *LEED for Homes Rating System* (2008). Washington, DC: U.S. Green Building Council. Available at: http://www.usgbc.org/ShowFile.aspx?DocumentID=3638. Accessed July 12, 2010.

Vigil, F. Black stains in houses: Soot, dust, or ghosts? *Home Energy Magazine*, January/February 1998.

Index

Insulation, 198–199
Insulation products
  caulks, 200
  combustion appliances, 199
  paint, 200
Integrated Pest Management (IPM), 38–39,
  104
International Code Council, 19, 152
International Energy Conservation Code
  (IECC), 156
International Property Maintenance Code
  (IPMC), 19, 152, 154
International Residential Code (IRC), 152,
  153
IPMC. *See* International Property
  Maintenance Code
IRC. *See* International Residential Code

J
Jerome meter, 107

K
Kitchens, 26

L
Laboratory testing, 105
  allergy testing, 107
  exposure to environmental tobacco
    smoke, 106
  exposure to heavy metals, 106
LaHouse, 144
Land-grant universities, 138–141
Lead, 197–198, 204–205
  paint, 21, 39, 95, 107, 153
  poisoning, 74, 78
Lead-based paint hazards, 16–17
Lead-contaminated dust, 28
Lead-contaminated paint, 28
Leaded paint ban in 1978, 16–17, 95, 106,
  197
Leadership in Energy and Environmental
  Design, 157

Lead hazards
  actions, 17
  strategies to control, 17
Lead-safe housing regulation, 128
Leaky homes, 192
  in cold climates, 193
Legislation and politics, 128
Local exhaust ventilation, 31
Low-income families
  eligible for the Weatherization Assistance
    Program, 192
Lung cancer, causes of, 105

M
Maintenance, 39–41
  limitations of, 45
  site, 44–45
Maintenance measures at home
  filtration change, 209
  spot ventilation, 209
Master Home Environmentalist Program, 125
Meals on Wheels Association of America
  (MOWAA), 174
Medical history, 94–95
Mercury exposures, 106
Metal sheets, 27
Methadone, 58
"Methodological pluralism," 10
Mid-level supervisors, 128
Mite allergens, 24. *See also* Allergens
Model energy codes, 155
Moisture, 21–22, 193
  household pests, 21
  levels in homes, measuring, 22–24
  meters, 23
  and mold remediation guidelines, 24
  prevention, 27
Moisture control
  and ventilation, 24–26
Mold, 24, 95, 104
  exposure, 21–22
  growth, 95, 99, 161

Mold (*continued*)
and moisture remediation guidelines, 24
sampling, 108
spores, 24
Mold-induced illnesses, 21
Morrill Acts, 138
MOWAA. *See* Meals on Wheels Association of America
Mycotoxins, 99

N
National Building Code, 151
National Center for Healthy Housing, 20, 95, 126, 143, 158
National Environmental Health Association, 20, 123
National Fire Alarm and Signaling Code, 174
National Fire Protection Association (NFPA), 166, 174
National Green Building Standard, 157
National Healthy Homes Training Center and Network, 20, 123, 126, 132, 143
National Public Health Leadership Development Network, 127
National Research Council 1993, 16
National Survey of Lead and Allergens in Housing, 21–22
Natural Resource Conservation Service, 142
Neural tube defects, 92
NFPA. *See* National Fire Protection Association
Nitrogen oxides, 193–194
Non-firefighters, training for, 185
Non-government resources
Association of Occupational and Environmental Clinics, 116
online resources, 116
Pediatric Environmental Health Specialty Units (PEHSUs), 112–116
poison-control centers, 116
working with other health professionals, 116

Norepinephrine
use by lower-income group, 19
North American Pediatric Environmental Health Specialty Units, 110–111

O
Older adults and housing needs, 9
Opioid pain medications, 58
Optimum value engineering, 159
Oxycodone, 58

P
Parents
training in basic lifesaving skills for, 62
Partnerships, types of, 185
Passive House Standard, 161
Patient evaluation, 91
critical windows of vulnerability, 92
Patients with building-related issues
examples of, 108–112
Pediatric Environmental Health Specialty Units (PEHSU), 110–111, 112
The Pediatric Environmental Home Assessment, 21
Pediatric Environmental Home Assessment Survey, 96–99
PEHSU. *See* Pediatric Environmental Health Specialty Units
Personal health workforce, 122
Pesticides, 29–30, 207
on male health, 92
residue testing, 107
storage, 104
Pest infestations, 30, 36
detection methods, 37–38
Integrated Pest Management (IPM), 38–39
Pets, 39
Physical examination of an individual, 105
Pitot tube, 32
Poison-control centers, 116
Poisonings, 57–58